MW00355845

# The
# Perinatal Nurse's Guide to
# Avoiding a Lawsuit

Patricia M. Connors,

RNC, MS, WHNP

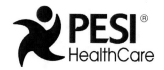

**PESI**®
HealthCare

PESI HealthCare
PO Box 900
Eau Claire, WI  54702-0900

Printed in the United States of America

ISBN: 0-9790218-6-3

PESI HealthCare strives to obtain knowledgeable authors and faculty for its publications and seminars. The clinical recommendations contained herein are the result of extensive author research and review. Obviously, any recommendations for patient care must be held up against individual circumstances at hand. To the best of our knowledge any recommendations included by the author or faculty reflect currently accepted practice. However, these recommendations cannot be considered universal and complete. The authors and publisher repudiate any responsibility for unfavorable effects that result from information, recommendations, undetected omissions or errors. Professionals using this publication should research other original sources of authority as well.

**For information on this and other PESI Healthcare educational products, please call 800-843-7763 or visit our website at www.pesihealthcare.com**

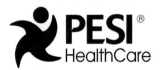

Cover photograph provided by Bob Bagwell

# About the Author

Patricia M. Connors, RNC, MS, WHNP, has over 40 years experience in perinatal nursing. She received both undergraduate and graduate degrees from Boston College in Chestnut Hill, Massachusetts and has held positions as a staff nurse, instructor of both undergraduate and graduate students, Women's Health Nurse Practitioner, nurse manager and clinical nurse specialist. She is presently a Perinatal Clinical Nurse Specialist at Massachusetts General Hospital in Boston, MA.

She is a member of Sigma Theta Tau International, the Association of Women's Health and Neonatal Nursing's Consulting Group and an AWHONN Fetal Heart Monitoring Principles and Practice Program Instructor. Publications include: "The Perinatal Nurse's Communication Responsibilities", Forum, March 2001, Vol 21; "High Risk Perinatal Issues: Failure to Recognize Fetal Distress and Insufficient Documentation" Journal of Nursing Law, May 2003, Vol 9 and "Shoulder Dystocia: Not a Second to Spare", Nursing Spectrum, January 2004, Vol. 8.

As a speaker for PESI HealthCare, she travels nationally presenting seminars addressing obstetrical errors and risk management. Her audience includes attorneys, risk managers, physicians and midwives as well as nurses.

# Table of Contents

Table of Contents

Table of Contents

# Dedication

To all the incredibly talented and dedicated perinatal nurses I have had the privilege of working with and learning from over the years. Because of the great care you render to mothers and babies on a daily basis, the good far outweighs the negative. Because of your dedication to your patients, tragedies are averted everyday and healthy mothers and babies are able to go home to start their lives. Let us never forget that it is so important that we remain vigilant of the need to continue improving patient safety so that no mother or baby will ever be harmed due to negligence, poor teamwork or lack of communication with our equally dedicated and talented physician, midwife, anesthesiologist and pediatric colleagues.

*P. M. C.*

# Forward

The transformation of nursing from a vocation to a profession has changed not only the practice of nursing, but also the vulnerability of the nurse as a target for medical malpractice suits. Gone are the days of blindly following the physician's orders. Gone are the days of rising from your seat when the surgeon enters the nurses' station. Gone are the days of having too few options available when giving patient care. Welcome are the days of college-prepared, highly skilled and specialized nurses. Welcome are the days of nurses who perform thorough assessments and use critical analysis skills when planning patient care. Welcome are the days of nurses working side by side with physicians and contributing to patient care with their own specific skill set and knowledge base. Nurses as professionals also have new-found responsibilities, commitments and accountability and are justifiably now held to a much higher standard than in years past.

As nursing became a profession, the law began to recognize the nurse as an accountable professional (with an insurance policy) and nurses joined physicians as co-defendants in medical malpractice lawsuits. Interestingly, the first nurses to be consistently added to medical malpractice actions were the obstetrical or perinatal nurses. This is a practice area that continues to see the most nurse defendants with emergency care nurses and critical care nurses coming in a somewhat distant second. Perinatal nursing has many rewards, but with those rewards, there is also the significant risk of being named in a lawsuit whenever the outcome for mother or baby is less than optimal. Some lawsuits are justified and some are not. Regardless, it has been my experience that nurses who are sued respond emotionally. They feel personally targeted. They feel guilty and question themselves as well as their actions. Many change the focus of their practice and no longer care for the laboring patient, or leave perinatal nursing all together. No matter the final outcome of the litigation, the nurse is injured, as is the entire profession.

The risk of litigation associated with the ever-satisfying practice of perinatal nursing must not deter us. Perinatal nurses must not seek new areas of specialization in the hope of avoiding litigation during their careers. Instead, perinatal nurses, as all nurses, must realize their new identity as professionals and meet the challenges of the professional status. Skills must be honed and lines of communications and relationships strengthened. Nursing must be constantly fed and nurtured with research incorporating new evidence into nursing standards of practice. And finally, risk management must be appreciated, taught and integrated into daily patient care. Only then will our daughters and future generations continue to have highly skilled and caring nurses assisting them during the birth of our children.

*Heather G. Beattie, RN, JD*

# Preface

My intention in writing The Perinatal Nurse's Guide to Avoiding a Lawsuit has been to share with colleagues my experiences and the knowledge I have acquired while working with both plaintiff and defense attorneys. It has been close to a decade now that I have been reviewing obstetrical cases for merit and testifying as an expert witness. While I am not an attorney (nor pretend to be one), I believe that I am in a unique position to educate nurses who care for mothers and newborns as to just what it is that might lead them to become involved in the dreaded LAWSUIT. I like to think of myself as a kind of Nancy Drew who has infiltrated "the other side" and can now bring the information back and help fellow perinatal nurses.

At one time, physicians were considered the "captain of the ship" and nurses were expected to do little more than take and follow orders. In fact, I still have attorneys who are surprised when I tell them that the role of the nurse has truly expanded and we are no longer "handmaidens". When I have an opportunity to enlighten an attorney, I also stress that we are actually well educated, autonomous and capable of critical thinking. Today's nurses may also find themselves responsible for many tasks once assigned to physicians. Unfortunately, it is not unheard of to have a nurse named in a lawsuit without the physician or midwife as co-defendant.

The maternal population has also changed and with that have come increased risks of complications. We now have older women choosing to have babies, the obesity issue is fraught with many potential complications and women who never would have thought of becoming pregnant are now doing so (i.e. cardiac patients, diabetics and those with cystic fibrosis, to name a few). Maternal-child nursing has become more complex with higher demands for assessment and vigilance so that both mother and newborn can be assured the best and safest care.

I have sought to highlight those areas of litigation that perinatal nurses are at greatest risk for and to address strategies to reduce those risks. I have also included many case studies. My intent is not to frighten, but to provide another venue from which to learn. The importance of the nursing process in caring for both mother and newborn, comprehensive and complete documentation, adherence to evidence based practice, the invaluable importance of working as a team, maintaining competencies, knowing how and when to initiate the chain of command and ingraining the ANA *Code of Ethics for Nurses* into our practice will be emphasized. Through all of this, the goal of high-quality patient care and the attainment of patient safety will be the focus.

I hope that you find my endeavor helpful in your practice and Chapter VIII totally useless!

*Patricia M. Connors, RNC, MS, WHNP*

# Code of Ethics for Nurses

*American Nurses Association*

1. The nurse in all relationships, practices with compassion and respect for the inherent dignity, worth, and uniqueness of every individual, unrestricted by considerations of social or economic status, personal attributes, or the nature of health problems.
2. The nurse's primary commitment is to the patient, whether an individual, family, group, or community.
3. The nurse promotes, advocates for, and strives to protect the health, safety, and rights of the patient.
4. The nurse is responsible and accountable for individual nursing practice and determines the appropriate delegation of tasks consistent with the nurse's obligation to provide optimum patient care.
5. The nurse owes the same duties to self as to others, including the responsibility to preserve integrity and safety, to maintain competence and to continue personal and professional growth.
6. The nurse participates in establishing, maintaining and improving health care environments and conditions of employment conducive to the provision of quality health care and consistent with the values of the profession through individual and collective action.
7. The nurse participates in the advancement of the profession through contributions to practice, education, administration and knowledge development.
8. The nurse collaborates with other health professionals and the public in promoting community, national and international efforts to meet health needs.
9. The profession of nursing, as represented by associations and their members, is responsible for articulating nursing values, for maintaining the integrity of the profession and its practice, and for shaping social policy.

# CHAPTER 1

# Why Errors Occur

*"Errors are made by highly competent, careful, and conscientious people for the simple reason that everyone makes mistakes every day. Thus, what we need to think about is not who is at fault or who is to blame, but why and how errors occur and, more importantly, what can be done to prevent them".*

*Dr. Lucian Leape*

Quality of care is a recurring theme within every nursing education program. From introductory to capstone courses, nurses learn and are expected to incorporate within their own practice high quality care that does not jeopardize patient safety.[1] To minimize patient harm and injury, it is important that perinatal nurses, physicians, nurse-midwives and others who care for women in the perinatal setting, be familiar with themes commonly associated with patient harm and accidents.[2]

---

**Did You Know?**

Between 44,000 and 98,000 patients die every year in hospitals because of errors by healthcare providers, more than because of traffic accidents, breast cancer, and human immunodeficiency virus infection, making these types of deaths the fourth leading cause of death in the United States.[3] These deaths include mothers and babies. Along with emergency departments and perioperative services, perinatal units account for most claims of patient injuries and deaths with fetal and neonatal being more common than maternal injuries. Many of the patient injuries related to human error are preventable.[4]

---

**Examples of Factors That May Contribute to Error**

**Environmental Factors**

- When appropriate resources are not available, patient care is placed in jeopardy. One of the unique features of perinatal nursing is the unpredictable patient volume that can occur and the unforeseen conditions that can make any low risk pregnant woman or neonate high risk. The nature of the unexpected can make even the best planned approach to staffing

substandard for any given day.[5]
- Inadequate staffing. Surveillance involves assessing patients frequently, attending to cues, and recognizing complications. When nurses are assigned to care for too many patients, their ability to monitor often and thoroughly and to "digest" recorded information may suffer. Novice nurses still honing their skills in patient care and time management will be particularly vulnerable, but an excessive patient load can overwhelm even the most experienced nurse.[6]
- A hostile environment in which doctors and nurses exhibit disruptive behavior. This is further explored in Chapter 2.
- Constant changes in today's healthcare system. (i.e., the shifting of more clinical care and technology to the ambulatory setting).

## Human Factors

- Fatigue: The IOM report *Keeping Patients Safe: Transforming the Work Environment of Nurses* recommended that nurses' work hours be regulated to not more than 12 hours in 24 hours and not more than 60 hours in 7 days.[7]
- Studies have shown that sleep deprivation and misalignment of the circadian rhythm phase as experienced during rotating shift work are each associated with frequent lapses of attention and increased reaction time, leading to increased error rates on performance tasks.[8]
  - ❖ The rate of medication errors increases after the 12th completed hour of work. In one study, 24 hours of sleep deprivation was equivalent to the performance with a blood alcohol level of 0.1%.[9, 10]
  - ❖ There is diminished ability to recognize subtle changes in a patient's condition.[11]
  - ❖ Leads to compromised critical thinking, problem solving, and decision making.[11]
  - ❖ Promotes reduced motivation leading to burnout.

---

**Did You Know?**

Nursing fatigue has been addressed by several organizations in an attempt to decrease nursing errors.

In 2005, the Association of periOperative Nurses (AORN) surveyed its members regarding on-call hours and effects. Among respondents, 77% routinely took call, 68% said that they had experienced sleep deprivation, 58% reported feeling unsafe while delivering patient care, and 13% reported making patient-care mistakes related to their fatigue. (Kenyon,T.,

---

Gluesing,R., White, K., Dunkel, W. & Burlingame, B. (2007). On call: Alert or unsafe? A report of the AORN On-call Electronic Task Force. AORN Journal, 86(4), 630-639.)

The Minnesota Nurses Association found that nurses are 3 times more likely to make errors if they work shifts longer than 12 hours per day or 60 hours per week. In addition to being more prone to making medical errors, nurses who work longer shifts experience more neck, shoulder, and back injuries than nurses who work 8-hour shifts. (Minnesota Nurses Association. (2007 January/February) #20 Nursing & fatigue. Minnesota Nursing Accent, 22-25.)

In 2008, The National Association of Neonatal Nurses (NANN) issued a Position Statement recommending education about fatigue be incorporated into nursing curriculum. NANN also recommends that all healthcare employers implement guidelines to minimize staff fatigue and that every RN should maintain awareness of his or her personal fatigue level because all RNs ultimately are responsible for their own practice. (The National Association of Neonatal Nurses. (2008). Position Statement #3044. Bedside Registered Staff Nurse Shift Length, Fatigue, and Impact on Patient Safety.)

- Inappropriate nursing assignment - the inexperienced nurse caring for the severe preeclamptic who is hesitant to ask for help for fear of looking incompetent.
- The novice nurse. We learn from experiences over time. The novice nurse has not had the benefit of building a library of experiences on which to rely. They need to use a procedurally driven process to make decisions, which is quite slow and prone to error. In contrast, the expert makes decisions by pattern matching. When they see a patient or a clinical situation, they have a large mental library of experience to match against. It is a rapid process and quite accurate if the expert continues to confirm the diagnosis against incoming information. For example, a patient presents to labor and delivery with a history of having been in a motor vehicle accident. She was not wearing a seat belt and hit her abdomen on the steering wheel. The expert would know that there is a danger of placental abruption and when the electronic monitor is placed on the patient would know what signs of fetal compromise to look for. The novice, since she has never been exposed to this scenario, might miss signs of uterine irritability and/or uteroplacental insufficiency.

- Illegible handwriting.
- Language differences.
- Multi-tasking - the mind becomes overloaded and unable to process all of the information it comes in contact with.
- Stress, which is known to actively degrade performance.
- Professional burnout which can impact an individual's empathy, energy, reaction time to emergencies and ability to concentrate.
- Normalization of Deviance

*Normalization of deviance* is an interesting concept which was first described by Vaughn in her analysis of the Challenger disaster.[12] According to this concept, people continue to perform unsafe tasks because "nothing ever happens." Overtime, these unsafe practices become part of the culture and ingrained in the everyday functioning of the unit. No one realizes that the standards of care are slowly becoming non-existent and being replaced by practices that carry a high potential for patient injury. Examples of normalization of deviance in perinatal care include:[4]

- ❖ Use of fundal pressure to shorten an otherwise normal second stage.
- ❖ Increasing oxytocin dosage administration during hyperstimulation.
- ❖ Performance of amniotomy with no indication when the fetus is at a high station.
- ❖ Application of a vacuum extractor using excessive pressures and timeframes.
- ❖ Aggressive, coached, closed-glottis pushing during the second stage with fetal heart rate decelerations.
- ❖ Not calling the neonatal resuscitation team when there is evidence of fetal compromise.
- ❖ Chronic understaffing.

An example of Normalization of Deviance that I can still remember very clearly happened 40 years ago when I was working as a staff nurse in labor and delivery. A patient of Dr. C's came into the hospital to deliver her fourth baby. She was in active labor. Dr C. sat at the end of her bed, ruptured her membranes and looked up at me and said, "I just prolapsed the cord. We need to go to the OR." All the way down the hall and throughout the surgery, I could hear Dr. C. mumbling to himself, "I've been doing this for 25 years and have never gotten caught." Well, he did get caught and the price was his patient required an otherwise unnecessary cesarean section.

Another example happened when an obstetrician I was assisting performed his usual ritual of winding up the umbilical cord on a Kelly clamp and tugging on the placenta after delivery of the baby. He did not like to wait for the normal separation of the placenta. Only this time, the uterus came with it. Thankfully, he was an experienced obstetrician and knew how to replace the uterus without having the patient loose too much blood or totally exsanguinate.

---

**Take Home Message**

We must remain vigilant and not let our guard down so that the care of mothers and newborns does not become "too routine" and it takes a tragedy to get us back on track.

---

## Patient Factors

- The patient does not give you all the information you need to care for her, such as allergies to certain medications or the fact that she was on bedrest for several weeks because of a bleeding episode when she was 5 months pregnant.

## Equipment/ Technology Factors

- The equipment is not programmed correctly or inservices have not been provided on new equipment. The following 2 cases illustrate the failure of nurses to determine the appropriate equipment to use for a specific patient or the appropriate use of equipment.

---

**Improper Use of Equipment**
Salter v. Deaconess Family Medical Center (1999)

On day 4 of life, Nurse Battaglia placed a wet washcloth on the heel of infant Demitrius Hawkins to help facilitate drawing blood. Prior to placing the cloth, she had heated it in a microwave for one minute. Nurse Battaglia testified that she had tested the cloth by touching it to her arm and it had felt satisfactory to her. The infant suffered second-degree burns that required various treatments, including debridement over a 3 month period. A law suit ensued and the nurse was found negligent.

In another case, a patient suffered significant burns to her back after the nurse applied a hot pack to her lower back during labor. The nurse had wrapped a wet towel in a blue chux pad and heated it in the microwave. The patient had epidural anesthesia and was not able to feel her skin burning. After delivery of her infant, the patient was discharged home, but had to return to the hospital's Burn Clinic for treatment. At this time, it is not known if a law suit has been filed.

---

# Why Errors Occur

## Systems Factors

The basic premise in the systems approach is that humans are fallible and errors are to be expected, even in the best organizations. Errors are seen as consequences rather than causes, having their origin not so much in the perversity of human nature as in "upstream" systemic factors. When an adverse event occurs, the important issue is not who blundered, but how and why the defenses (error traps) which were thought to be effective and in place, failed.[13]

The greatest contributor to errors, according to Dr. Lucian Leape, is the design of the underlying system and the organizational practices and culture. The mistake or error is a signal that there is something wrong.[14] Dr. Leape's research has helped shift conventional thinking away from blaming individuals when errors occur to focusing on the systems as a source of the problem.[15] Accidents are not caused by individuals, but rather, produced by gaps and vulnerabilities contained within the imperfect system and organizations in which health care is delivered.[16] Thus, mistakes can best be prevented by designing the health system at all levels to make it safer - to make it harder for people to do something wrong and easier for them to do it right. This does not mean that individuals can be careless. People still need to be vigilant and held responsible for their actions. But when an error occurs, blaming an individual does little to make the system safer and prevent someone else from committing the same error.[17]

Human-factors specialists describe complex systems like health-care organizations as inverted pyramids. The broad blunt end on top consists of managers, administrators, and regulators: the people who set the policies and enforce the rules. Doctors and nurses are at the sharp end of the pyramid, interacting directly with patients. Their mistakes are more obvious because they usually have immediate, often serious, consequences. Accident investigations reveal consistently that the ability of the people at the sharp end to prevent adverse incidents depends on a host of factors determined at the blunt end, rather than isolated acts of one individual.[18] Reason[19] describes defense layers that are put in place by organizations in attempt to barricade errors as Swiss cheese: full of holes. Such holes exist in all complex hazardous systems because the decision makers cannot foresee all of the possible accident scenarios. The slices of cheese represent successive layers of defenses, barriers and safeguards, but when the holes are lined up just right, accidents can and do occur. These gaps and failures occur for two reasons:

- Active failures: described as unsafe acts on the part of those in direct contact with the patient or system (sharp end of the pyramid).
- Latent conditions: these are defensive gaps, weaknesses or absences that are unwittingly created as the result of earlier decisions made by the de-

signers, builders, regulators, and managers of the system. (blunt end of the pyramid). Latent failures create the possibilities and probabilities for active failures.

According to Reason[19], the two questions that need to be asked after an organizational accident are first, "How did each defense or barrier fail?" and secondly, "Why did it fail?"

The systems concept has been very difficult for both the nursing and medical communities to grasp as the prevention of errors has historically been viewed as an individual problem and when they do occur, punitive action may be taken. The health care system is locked into a paradigm of preventing errors by training people very highly, holding them to high standards, and expecting people to make no mistakes. The concept of "train and blame" exists and errors are not to be tolerated.[14, 20] Equally important is the legal system and its role in promoting cultures of fear and blame, especially in perinatal care. The nature of tort law is punitive, resulting in monetary damages being paid by any party found liable.[21]

**Loss of Situational Awareness**

Situational awareness is a shared understanding of "what's going on" and "what is likely to happen next."[22] Situational awareness allows us to recognize events around us, act correctly when things proceed as planned, and react appropriately when they do not. Loss of situational awareness is a precursor of error, bad judgment or the patient harm that results from the perinatal team's inability to recognize, mitigate or recover once an error has occurred, that is, an indication that something is wrong or about to go wrong.[2]

---

**Example of Loss of Situational Awareness and Communication[23]**

At 41 weeks of an uneventful pregnancy, Mrs. W arrived at Beth Israel Deaconess Medical Center in Boston, Massachusetts, one night in November 2000. Sometime before 10 p.m. an exam revealed her cervix to be closed and she was given a drug to induce labor. At 10 p.m., she was sent home. On the way home, she began to experience contractions, became very uncomfortable and returned to the hospital. She was admitted to the hospital at midnight, contracting every 1-2 minutes and vomiting. At 4:30 a.m., the fetal heart rate showed an unusual ''sawtooth'' pattern and her cervix was dilated 4 to 5 centimeters. At 5:50-5:53, the fetal heart rate dropped to 90 beats per minute and continued to slow until 6:04.

---

> At 6:20, delivery was attempted with forceps but was not successful and the patient was transferred to the operating room for a cesarean section. A stillborn 10 pound male was delivered at 6:45 a.m. Mrs. W. also required a hysterectomy for refractory uterine atony, developed ARDS, DIC and sepsis. She spent 3 weeks in the hospital before being transferred to a rehabilitation center.

When a Root Cause Analysis was done, it showed numerous failures in communication, situational awareness and planning which included:

- The staff caring for Mrs. W. were not vigilant of the changes occurring.
- Mrs. W. should never have been discharged due to her blood pressure being 124/90 at discharge and upon returning to the hospital it was 174/104. No one considered preecalmpsia and no plan was formulated.
- The cesarean section should have been performed at 5:30 a.m. for nonreassuring FHR and if there was to be trial of forceps, it should have been done in the operating room to save precious time.
- In the 5 ½ hours prior to delivery, there were 12 assessments done but no clear clinical plan communicated to all staff and to the patient. There was very little documentation.
- The nurse caring for Mrs. W. was new, had never seen a "sawtooth" pattern and was not being supervised by a more experienced nurse due to the unit being extremely busy. The fetal heart rate patterns were not appreciated.
- The physician had been working 21 hours straight and showed "vigilance fatigue."

In response to this very tragic event, the Beth Israel Deaconess Hospital instituted several changes including team training. In 2001, Harvard's Risk Management Foundation, the Armed Forces Institute of Pathology, the Office of the Assistant Secretary of Defense (Health Affairs), and Dynamics Research Corporation approached the department to adapt concepts of team training to obstetrics. The communication issues laid bare by Mrs. W's case suggested that team training could potentially help the staff address issues of communication, cross-monitoring, mutual support, situational awareness, conflict resolution, and variable workload.[23]

**Ineffective Communication**

> **Did You Know?**
>
> Ineffective communication was cited as the root cause of 66% of all reported sentinel events from 1995 to 2004 and accounted for 85% of sentinel events related to maternal death and injury in 2005.
>
> http://www.jointcommission.org/sentinel events/statistics

Communication problems are consistently identified as a leading cause of system breakdown in patient care.[2, 17, 24, 25] In July 2004, the Joint Commission on Accreditation of Healthcare Organizations issued a Sentinel Event Alert targeting the significant contribution of communication problems to potentially preventable perinatal morbidity and mortality.[26]

Part of the problem is that physicians and nurses communicate differently. Nurses are trained to be narrative and descriptive while physicians want the headlines. "What's the problem? What's the fix?" When a nurse speaks to a physician, he/she expects "JUST THE FACTS, MA'AM." When too much extraneous information is given, the provider can loose sight of what it is exactly that the nurse is trying to convey. SBAR, which will be discussed in Chapter 2, is one method that addresses this mismatch of communication.

---

**Example of Ambiguous Communication**
**Wingo v. Rockford Memorial Hospital (1997)**

Mrs. Wingo, at term, was admitted to the hospital with an initial rupture of membranes and irregular contractions. The physician examined the patient early in the day and, noting no fluid, assumed either her membranes had not ruptured or had sealed over. However, the nurse caring for the patient had assessed amniotic fluid continuing to leak from the patient all day and the onset of regular contractions. When the physician called the nurse caring for Mrs. Wingo to inquire about her condition, the nurse reported "no change" in her condition. The physician believed that the patient had stabilized and that it was safe to discharge her. Later that night, Mrs. Wingo delivered a baby girl who had exhibited signs of fetal distress and now is neurologically impaired.

The court concluded that the nurse must take responsibility for reporting a patient's condition in a manner that will be understood by the physician. "No change in condition" could have different meanings, depending on the perspective of the person observing the patient. The nurse needs to be clear when communicating information that may influence the decisions the provider makes when formulating a plan of care.

---

1.  Maddox P, Wakefield M, Bull J. Patient safety and the need for professional and educational change. *Nursing Outlook.* 2001;49:8-13.
2.  Simpson KR, Knox GE. Adverse perinatal outcomes: Recognizing, understanding & preventing common accidents. *AWHONN Lifelines.* 2003; 7:225-235.
3.  To err is human: Building a safer health system. Washington DC: National Academy of Science; 1999.
4.  Simpson K, Creehan P. *Perinatal Nursing.* 2nd ed. Philadelphia: Lippincott; 2001.
5.  Rostant D, Cady R. *Liability Issues in Perinatal Nursing.* Philadelphia: Lippincott; 1999.
6.  Clarke SP, Aiken LH. Failure to rescue: Needless deaths are prime examples of the need for more nurses at the bedside. *Am J Nurs.* 2003;103:42-47.
7.  Page A, ed. *Keeping Patients Safe:Transforming the Work Environment of Nurses.* Washington, DC: National Academies Press; 2004.
8.  Gold DR, Rogacz S, Bock N, et al. Rotating shift work, sleep, and accidents related to sleepiness in hospital nurses. *Am J Public Health.* 1992;82:1011-1014.
9.  Gaba DM, Howard SK. Patient safety: Fatigue among clinicians and the safety of patients. *N Engl J Med.* 2002;347:1249-1255.
10. Rogers AE, Hwang WT, Scott LD, Aiken LH, Dinges DF. The working hours of hospital staff nurses and patient safety. *Health Aff (Millwood).* 2004;23:202-212.
11. Pastorius D. Crime in the workplace, part 1. *Nurs Manage.* 2007;38:18-27.
12. Vaughn D. *The Challenger Launch Decision: Risky Technology, Culture and Deviance at NASA.* Chicago: University of Chicago Press; 1996.
13. Reason J. Human error: Models and management. *BMJ.* 2000;320:768-770.
14. Buerhaus PI. Lucian Leape on the causes and prevention of errors and adverse events in health care. *Image J Nurs Scholarsh.* 1999;31:281-286.
15. Buerhaus PI. Lucian Leape on patient safety in U.S. hospitals... includes discussion. *J Nurs Scholarsh.* 2004;36:366-370.
16. Vincent C, ed. *Clinical Risk Management.* 2nd ed. London: BMJ Books; 2001. Reason JT, ed. Understanding Adverse Events: The Human Factor.
17. Institute of Medicine. To err is human. Washington, DC: National Academies Press; 2000.
18. MacReady N. Second stories, sharp ends: Dissecting medical errors. *Lancet.* 2000;355:994-996.
19. Reason J. Beyond the organizational accident: The need for "error wisdom" on the frontline. *Qual Safe Health Care.* 2004;13:28-33.

20. Buerhaus PI. Follow-up conversation with Lucian Leape on errors and adverse events in health care. *Nurs Outlook.* 2001;49:73-77.

21. Miller LA. Safety promotion and error reduction in perinatal care: Lessons from industry. *J Perinat Neonat Nurs.* 2003;17:128-138.

22. Stanton N, Chambers P, Piggott J. Situational awareness and safety. *Safety Science.* 2001;39:189-204.

23. Sachs B. A 38 year old woman with fetal loss and hysterectomy. *JAMA.* 2005;294:833-840.

24. Institute of Medicine. Keeping patients safe: Transforming the work environment of nurses. Washington DC: National Academies Press; 2004.

25. Institute of Medicine. Crossing the quality chasm: A new health system for the 21st century. Washington DC: National Academies Press; 2001.

26. Joint Commission on Accreditation of Healthcare Organizations. Preventing infant death and injury during delivery. 2004;Sentinel Event Alert #30:1-3.

# CHAPTER 2

# Creating a Culture of Safety

*One of the first steps in the process of creating a safer health care system is to promote a culture of safety within the organization. A culture of safety is one in which individuals are encouraged to report error; therefore the system, not the individual, is assessed.[1]*

The Institute of Medicine's (IOM) landmark report, 'To Err is Human: Building a Safer Health System,"[2] carried four core messages; first, the magnitude of harm that results from medical errors is great; second, errors result largely from systems failures, not individual failures; third, voluntary and mandatory reporting programs are needed to improve patient safety; and fourth, the IOM committee and others call on health systems to focus on error reduction as an important part of their operations and to embrace organizational change needed to reorient error-ridden systems and process.[3] The Institute of Medicine lifted the veil on health care's most prevalent culture, the culture of *secrecy*. In forcing us to admit that "to err is human," researchers and the bright lights of the media opened the door for us to begin addressing errors more systematically.[4]

In 2001, the IOM published *Crossing the Quality Chasm: A New Health System for the 21st Century*, which is a report designed to guide efforts to improve the healthcare system. The IOM describes healthcare as a need to be:[5]

❑ **Safe**: Patients should not be harmed by the care that is intended to help them.

❑ **Effective**: Care should be based on scientific knowledge and offered to all who could benefit, and not to those not likely to benefit.

❑ **Patient-Centered**: Care should be respectful of and responsive to individual patient preferences, needs and values.

❑ **Timely**: Waiting and, sometimes harmful delays in care, should be reduced both for those who receive care and those who give care.

❑ **Efficient**: Care should be given without wasting equipment, supplies, ideas, and energy.

❑ **Equitable**: Care should not vary in quality because of personal characteristics such as gender, ethnicity, geographic location, and socio-economic status.

## The Nurse's Role in Error Reduction

Nurses play a key role in the national agenda of error reduction in healthcare because they are present most continuously with patients, and maintain a tradition of advocacy. Nurses daily monitor and manage the quality of healthcare delivered in hospitals, outpatient departments, long-term care facilities, and many other settings.[6] They play a key role in detecting and preventing errors, yet, unfortunately, are not immune.

## Near Misses and Good Catches

Evidence suggests that, on average, four latent errors precede and/or are coincident with every medical accident.[7] It is virtually impossible for one person or one error to be solely responsible when a mistake leads to patient injury. The critical issue is to have systems in place to catch the error before it results in an adverse outcome.[8] Perinatal units, like other high-risk, high-technology organizations, operate with many built in defense mechanisms that work to prevent errors from occurring. Maintaining appropriate staffing levels, the credentialing of health care providers, proper training of staff, and individual accountability for competency are only a few examples of these defenses against error, which form what can be conceptualized as multiple layers of protection against accident or error.[9]

However, it would take an extremely rare system not to have some vulnerabilities and the potential to be infiltrated. It has been suggested that professionals create safety at the point of care by routinely recognizing and recovering from the continuous array of errors produced by imperfect systems. These are the "good catches" or "near misses" that do not result in patient injury. Good catches imply vigilance, awareness, critical thinking, prompt action, and patient advocacy.[10]

---

**Examples of the Importance of Reporting Near Misses and Good Catches**

#1 A hospital pharmacy began stocking the labor and delivery unit with look-alike amber ampoules of 2 different drugs. One ampoule contained a tocolytic used for intrauterine resuscitation, and the other contained a strong uterotonic given to treat post partum hemorrhage. The nursing staff was not aware of the change. The drugs were placed next to each other in

---

the same drawer of the labor and delivery cart by a nursing assistant assigned to stock carts. Shortly thereafter, Nurse A. was preparing to administer a tocolytic per protocol, for a prolonged fetal heart rate deceleration during labor. She picked up an amber vial (usually the tocolytic was the only amber ampoule in the drawer), and prepared to administer the drug. A second nurse, Nurse B., picked up the opened ampoule to discard it and noticed that the nurse had inadvertently drawn up the uterine stimulant. Nurse B. averted a sure disaster by stopping Nurse A. from administering the wrong drug.

Since no harm was done, Nurse A. did not plan to write an incident report, but to report the problem to her nurse manager. Nurse B., who was the charge nurse, instructed Nurse A. to complete an incident report. She also consulted with the unit manager and pharmacy, and the uterotonic drug was immediately removed from the carts and placed in another accessible location.

Source: Mahlmeister, L. (2006). Best practices in perinatal care: Reporting "near misses" and "good catches" as a risk reduction strategy. *Journal of Perinatal and Neonatal Nursing*, 20 (3): 197-199.

#2   While giving discharge instructions to a postpartum patient with the assistance of an Arabic interpreter via a telephone service, the patient's husband (who spoke and understood English) brought it to the attention of the nurse that the interpreter was not giving the same instructions that the nurse was saying. Upon learning this, the nurse terminated the conversation and filled out a Safety Report. The Safety Report was followed up by the hospital's Interpreter Service Department and the following ensued:

- The account manager of the company providing the services met with the interpreter in question who admitted that what the nurse said was indeed true and that she was not as alert as she should have been due to feeling ill that day.
- A plan was set forth that the interpreter would be suspended from her interpreting duties for a time and when they were reinstated, all her calls would be monitored.

One can only imagine what harm could have happened had the nurse not reported this incident and the interpreter continued to give instructions to patients with more serious conditions (i.e., explaining surgery to a patient, or instructing them on taking medications such as insulin or Lovenox.)

Reporting near misses provides opportunity to openly analyze and discuss situations in a congenial, non accusatory environment in which team members do not feel threatened since patient harm has not occurred. It is an opportune time to commend them for having averted a potentially poor outcome, to emphasize the benefits of reporting "near misses and "good catches" and to encourage them to continue their commitment to patient safety.

**Error Detection**

*There are some patients we cannot help; there are none we cannot harm.*
*Arthur Bloomfield, MD*

Perhaps the most distinguishing feature of high reliability organizations (systems operating in hazardous conditions that have fewer than their fair share of adverse events) is their collective preoccupation with the possibility of failure. They expect to make errors and train their workforce to recognize and recover from them. They continually rehearse familiar scenarios of failure and strive hard to imagine novel ones. Instead of isolating failures, they generalize them. Instead of making local repairs, they look for system reforms. Individuals may forget to be afraid, but the culture of a high reliability organization provides them with both the reminders and tools to help them remember.[11]

The types and frequencies of reported errors are a function of the method of detection. A commonly used method is to review charts and interview care providers. Anonymous reporting may also be used, but cannot provide incidence because the reporting is voluntary; however, anonymous provider reporting is particularly useful for identifying rare and latent potential hazards.[12] Traditionally, incident reporting at the individual unit level has been the method that was used to identify harm to patients, but these are only partially successful. Reasons include: fear of a punitive response, lack of available time, cumbersome reporting methods, lack of prompt feedback and failure of the report to generate change.[12] The primary purpose of reporting is to learn from experience. It is based on actual practice which provides an insight into those areas of practice that are in need of improvement. Many other methods are also used to identify threats to safety, but a good internal reporting system ensures that all responsible parties are aware of major hazards. Reporting is also important for monitoring progress in the prevention of errors.[13]

**Frequency of Medication Errors in a NICU as Detected by Chart Review and Care Provider Interviews[14]**

In one NICU study, medication errors were found to be frequent (91 per 100 admissions) and more likely associated with the potential for harm than medication errors in infants, older children, and adults. Medication errors occurred most frequently in dosing (28%), followed by route of administration (18%), transcription and documentation (14%), date (12%), and frequency of administration (9%). The stage at which the error occurred most commonly was at the physician ordering stage, both for all errors (74%) and for those with potential to harm (79%). Physician reviewers concluded that 93% of the potential adverse drug events (ADEs) were preventable by the presence of a ward-based-clinical pharmacist.

**Table 2-1** lists the characteristics that have been identified as essential for a successful reporting program.

### Table 2-1 Characteristics of Successful Reporting Systems[13]

| Characteristic | Explanation |
| --- | --- |
| Non-punitive | Reporters are free of fear of retaliation or punishment from others as a result of reporting. |
| Confidential | The identities of the patient, reporter, and institution are never revealed to a third party. |
| Independent | The program is independent of any authority with power to punish the reporter or organization. |
| Expert Analysis | Reports are evaluated by experts who understand the clinical circumstances and who are trained to recognize underlying systems causes. |
| Timely | Reports are analyzed promptly, and recommendations are rapidly disseminated to those who need to know, especially when serious hazards are identified. |
| Systems oriented | Recommendations focus on changes in systems, processes, or products, rather than on individual performance. |
| Responsive | The agency that receives reports is capable of disseminating recommendations, and participating organizations agree to implement recommendations when possible. |

---

**Take Home Message**

Once all staff members witness that the culture provides a safe haven for admitting to, correcting, and learning from errors, they will begin to report their own errors. The goal is to make safety everyone's responsibility.[15]

---

**Sentinel Events and Root Cause Analysis**

In 1999, the Joint Commission on Accreditation of Healthcare Organizations (JCAHO) began requiring health facilities to conduct a Root Cause Analysis (RCA) for all sentinel events. A sentinel event is an unexpected occurrence involving death or serious physical or psychological injury, or the risk there of. "Sentinel" is used because it signals the need for immediate investigation and response. It is estimated that hospitals experience 10-20 sentinel events each year.[1] Examples of Sentinel Event Alerts specific to perinatal care include: infant abduction, high alert medications such as Magnesium sulfate, delays in treatment (Cesarean sections), perinatal deaths and Kernicterus.

The process for a Root Cause Analysis is described as:
- Focusing on systems and not individuals
- The process should ask "Why?"
- Thorough and credible
- Leadership is involved as well as those most closely involved
- There must be an explanation of all findings
- At the end of the process, an action plan and risk reduction strategies complete with timeframes and an appointed responsible person are implemented

The foundation for delivering safer perinatal and neonatal care is promoting a supportive culture of reporting errors and "near misses" or "good catches." The RCA is an ideal process in that it brings health care professionals together so that they may identify systems problems, come to a solution together and work as a team in implementing the agreed upon risk reduction strategies. Hierarchy should not enter into decisions and all should have an equal voice at the table. By keeping the patient as the main focus, care can be improved and injuries avoided.

It must also be remembered that not all sentinel events are the result of errors. For example, a maternal death, though unexpected, may be unavoidable if the woman suddenly develops an amniotic fluid embolism or deteriorates as a result of consumptive coagulopathy. An infant weighing more than 2,500 g may not survive a complete placental abruption or prolapsed cord. The key issue is to carefully analyze the event with the goal of developing strategies to prevent future occurrences.[16]

---

**Did You Know?**

**The Federal Patient Safety Task Force** was established in April 2001 within the Department of Health and Human Services to coordinate a joint effort among several department agencies to improve existing systems to collect data on patient safety. The task force was charged with working closely with the states and private sector to develop data to help avert risks to patients. The goal of this Task Force is to identify the data that healthcare providers, states, and others need to collect to improve patient safety. The agencies include the:

- Agency for Healthcare Research and Quality (AHRQ)
- Centers for Disease Control and Prevention (CDC)
- Food and Drug Administration (FDA)
- Center for Medicare and Medicaid Services(CMS) formerly known as Health Care Financing Administration (HCFA)

---

**Teamwork**

*Talent wins games, but teamwork and intelligence win championships.*
*Michael Jordan*

The aviation industry has long understood the importance of teamwork in accident and error avoidance. Organizational problems, errors by personnel, and poor teamwork were cited as causes related to aircraft accidents as early as 1951.[17] In response to these causes, Crew Resource Management (CRM), a structured program, was developed and addresses: attention management, crew management (communication and teamwork), stress management, attitude management, and risk management. Today, CRM programs are the norm in military and commercial aviation.[17] The success the aviation industry has had with team driven safety models was cited in the Institute of Medicine's follow-up report, *Crossing the Chasm.*[5] The report recommended that teamwork be focused on since labor and delivery units are high risk environments in which decisions must be made quickly, with care coordinated between multiple disciplines (obstetrics, nursing, anesthesia and neonatology) much the same as the airline industry.

The world of medicine has long been of the mindset that we are trained to be individual experts. Currently, in most labor and delivery units, patient information is not shared in a coordinated way between providers. When there is a shift change, for instance, nurses sign out to nurses, obstetricians hand off patients to obstetricians (often by phone or e-mail), residents attend teaching rounds, and rarely are anesthesiologists and neonatologists included in any sign-out of important information regarding OB patients.[18]

However, now, because of the increased complexity of care, we need to accept that we are working in an environment that often will surpass our individual capabilities. There is a need to work collectively, talk together and have a common vision. In any situation requiring a real time combination of multiple skills, experiences, and judgment, teams - as opposed to individuals - create superior performance.[16]

## What Teamwork Is and Is Not

Teamwork is a set of interrelated behaviors, cognitions and attitudes. Skill and knowledge are combined with the ability to anticipate the needs of each of the team members. Team members work in sync and are able to recognize potential problems or dangerous circumstances and adjust their strategies under stress. When deviations in normal procedures occur, medical team members must be able to adapt to the dynamic nature of the situation.[15]

Team members trust each other and, therefore, communicate well. Teamwork is not the sharing of the "group hug" or an "exclusive club," but a shared goal of vigilance to ensure patient safety. Teams do not always need to remain the same and can be flexible in their members.

Individual performance monitoring is essential to teamwork in that it allows team members to act as a second or third pair of eyes and ears by monitoring each other in an effort to catch mistakes, slips, or lapses prior to, or shortly after, they have occurred. However, in order for performance monitoring to be accepted by individuals it must be made clear that the purpose is to improve performance and patient safety, rather than to keep a record of mistakes for negative intentions. The focus should be on continuous improvement and development, not administrative or punitive.[15] All members must buy into this concept for the common good of the team.

---

**Take Home Message**

Anything done at the level of excellence, or in the pursuit of excellence, is exciting and fun. Anything done at the level of mediocrity is discouraging and a real drag. Where there is low morale, we often make low pay or hard work the scapegoats. However, I suspect it is more often the

---

dispiriting effect of poor team performance, finger-pointing negativity, and uninspired leadership. The best way I know to break this vicious cycle of poor performance that leads to low morale, that leads to poor performance, is to inspire a team to become better and better in an area they all believe is important.

*Fred Lee, If Disney Ran Your Hospital,*
*9 1/2 Things You Would Do Differently*

## TeamSTEPPS

TeamSTEPPS, a trademark of the Agency for Healthcare Research and Quality and the Department of Defense, is an evidence-based framework used to optimize team performance across the healthcare delivery system. It is comprised of four teachable-learnable skills:

1. *Leadership*, which is defined as the ability to coordinate the activities of team members by ensuring team actions are understood, changes in information are shared, and that team members have the necessary resources. Effective team leaders are essential and are able to organize the team, articulate clear goals, make decisions through collective input of members, empower members to speak up and challenge when appropriate, actively promote and facilitate good teamwork and skillfully address conflict resolution.

2. *Situation monitoring*, defined as the process of actively scanning and assessing situational elements to gain information, understanding, or maintaining awareness to support functioning of the team. It is knowing "what is going on around you" and having all the team members "on the same page." Components of situation monitoring include:

   **S**tatus of the patient
   - Patient history
   - Vital signs
   - Medications
   - Physical exam
   - Plan of Care
   - Psychosocial

   Assessment of the Level of **T**eam Members'
   - Fatigue
   - Workload
   - Task performance
   - Skill
   - Stress

Assessment of the **E**nvironment
- Facility information
- Administrative information
- Human resources
- Triage acuity
- Equipment

Assessment of the **P**rogress Towards the Goal
- Status of Team's Patient(s)?
- Established goals of the team
- Tasks/actions of team
- Is the plan of care still appropriate?

3. *Mutual support*, which is the ability to anticipate and support other team members' needs through accurate knowledge about their responsibilities and workload. Mutual support is evidenced when team members protect each other from work overload situations, all offers and requests for assistance are placed in the context of patient safety and team members foster a climate where it is expected that assistance will be actively *sought* and *offered*.

4. *Communication*, which is defined as the process by which information is clearly and accurately exchanged among team members. SBAR is a technique for communicating critical information that requires immediate attention and action concerning a patient's condition.

---

**What is SBAR?**

SBAR is a structured or effective communication tool that states the <u>S</u>ituation, <u>B</u>ackground, <u>A</u>ssessment, and <u>R</u>ecommendation. Use of the tool allows team members to organize their thoughts clearly, and concisely present them to another team member.

*<u>S</u>ituation - the punch line in 5-10 seconds

    Identify yourself and where you are calling from

    Patient's name and reason for report

    Patient was admitted for_____

    I am concerned about:

        FHR

        Contraction pattern

        Blood pressure

        Vaginal bleeding

*<u>B</u>ackground - the context, objective data, how did we get here

    Gravida____ Para_____ @_____weeks gestation

    OB or CNM attending_____

    Significant medical and OB history

---

Problems with current pregnancy are_____

Relate the complaints of the patient

*Assessment - what is the problem?

    Maternal vital signs

    FH= Baseline, Variability, Accelerations, Decelerations, Contraction Pattern (Using NICHD terminology)

    Significant Lab Values

    Intrauterine Resuscitative Measures

    Give your conclusions about the present situation.

*Recommendation - what do we need to do?

    What I need from you is_____

    Be specific about a time frame

    Suggestions for tests/treatments/medications

    Clarify orders, vital sign frequency, under what circumstances to call back

SBAR not only ensures that everyone gets what they want, but also helps develop critical thinking: when people pick up the phone, they have this model in their mind of what they actually have to deliver. SBAR is an effective bridge for a group of people who interact all day long, but who are trained to communicate differently.[19]

Poor communication among team members regarding the plan of care for a patient is a common path for substandard care. Assertive communication has been shown to be the key to maintaining safe operations. To be effective, it is important to understand the attributes of appropriate assertive communication; that it is not aggressive, hostile, confrontational, ambiguous or ridiculing. By contrast, being appropriately assertive means:[8]

- Being organized in thought and communication
- Being technically and socially competent
- Disavowing perfection while looking for clarification and/or common understudying
- Being owned by the entire team

The phrase "I am concerned" should rally all team members' attention so that all aspects of the patient's care is reassessed and loss of situational awareness is curtailed.

Case Example: Dysfunctional Teamwork
http://www.rmf.harvard.edu/case-studies

Clinical Sequence (of the case example)

In the 41st week of her first pregnancy, 38-year-old Tina Constanople (not her real name) arrived at labor and delivery for a planned induction of labor. Her pregnancy had progressed normally until the last month of her third trimester, when her blood pressure began to increase. She was diagnosed as having mild pregnancy-induced hypertension that responded to reduced activity and bed rest. At her 40 week visit, her cervix was found to be long and closed, her blood pressure was slightly elevated but stable, and she had +1 Proteinuria. Plans were made for induction of labor.

6:45 a.m.  Tina had intra-vaginal placement of Misoprostol. The nurse observed her briefly and then, at 11 a.m., Tina was discharged from the unit and went for a walk.

12:00 noon  Tina's membranes spontaneously ruptured and she returned to the Labor and Delivery unit. The nurse, a recently hired new graduate, admitted Tina to a labor room, took her vital signs and checked the fetal heart rate. Tina's blood pressure was 176/95; the nurse attributed this to her nausea, vomiting and discomfort from contractions.

12:10 p.m.  The resident on duty examined Tina and determined that her cervix was 5-6 cm, 90 percent effaced, and the vertex was at 0 station. A scalp electrode was placed and the fetal heart rate was recorded as 120 with no decelerations.

2:05 p.m.  Following painful contractions, Tina requested an epidural. After placement of the epidural, the monitor indicated a prolonged fetal heart rate deceleration. The heart rate returned slowly to the baseline rate of 120 as the nurse repositioned Tina, increased her intravenous fluids, and administered oxygen by mask.

2:15 p.m.  An epidural analgesia infusion pump was started. The fetal heart rate strip indicated another deceleration that recovered to baseline. The nurse informed the resident who checked the strip and told her to "keep an eye on things."

2:45 p.m.  The primary nurse noted in the labor record that the baseline fetal heart rate was, "unstable, between 100-120;" she did not report this to the resident.

3:05 p.m.  As the nurse recorded that the fetal heart rate was "nonreassuring: flat, no variability," the patient expressed a strong urge to push. The nurse called for an exam.

3:20 p.m.  A second resident came to the bedside, examined Tina, and noted that she was fully dilated with the caput at +1. A brief update was written in the chart but not initialed.

3:30 p.m.  Tina was repositioned and started pushing.

4:05 p.m.    The fetal heart rate suddenly dropped and remained profoundly bradycardic for 11 minutes. The resident was called and, since the fetal head was at +2 station, attempted a vacuum delivery. The attending then entered and attempted forceps delivery.

4:35 p.m.    An emergency cesarean delivery was performed, but the baby was stillborn. The physician identified a uterine rupture that required significant blood replacement.

A medical malpractice claim was filed against two attendings, two obstetric residents, and the primary nurse. The plaintiffs claimed that a serious fetal heart rate pattern was either unrecognized or misinterpreted. They further alleged that the FHR changes (loss of variability, decelerations and bradycardia) should have prompted a more aggressive delivery strategy. The claim was settled in excess of $1 million.

Discussion Points

1. Junior members of the mother's care team, in this case a nurse and physician, shied away from voicing their concerns or challenging decisions made by more senior clinicians. *All members of the care team should be encouraged to speak up if they disagree with a management plan or they are seriously concerned about their patient's care. All members should be equally heard and their opinions valued. When there is a disagreement with a management decision, there should be a clearly defined way of resolving the conflict. All staff members should be knowledgeable of the Chain of Command.*

2. At least six individuals were involved in this patient's care over the nine hours following Induction - 2 attendings, 2 residents, a primary nurse and at least 1 to 2 other nurses. *Achieving a good clinical outcome requires effective communication, coordination among all the care givers involved, with adequate documentation of the management plan. When everyone involved shares a common set of behaviors and routinely brief, share and review clinical information in a timely fashion, then there are greater opportunities to ensure safe patient care.*

3. Although the care team responded to the fetal bradycardia, there was no indication that other resources were promptly alerted to the emerging crisis. *The impact of certain clinical events or information often extends beyond the obvious problem. A situation that demands greater monitoring may impact staffing, thus the resource nurse should know about it. All essential disciplines*

*should be aware of the potential need for emergency help - anesthesia, NICU - before a crisis arises.*

4. The fact that the fetus had a "nonreassuring" heart rate tracing was not shared among team members and the situation was not promptly addressed. The record made no mention of intrauterine resuscitative efforts. When the situation eventually became a critical, the care team was insufficiently prepared. *The defense of care provided during a crisis benefits from evidence (i.e. documentation) that the providers a) were prepared for contingencies, and b) followed an established protocol once things became emergent. The absence of such evidence leaves patients and jurors to conclude otherwise.*

## Communication Handoffs

Adverse medical events are frequently the result of ineffective team communication: either not having enough information, loosing it across the transitions of care, or one clinician having a different "picture" of what's supposed to be done than others caring for the same patient. Multiple people caring for a given patient need a systematic process to facilitate communication and keep everyone in the same "movie."[19]

The patient report is an important part of the communication processes which take place within the nurse's working day. The most conservative estimate of nurse hours devoted to handover report each day is seven, the equivalent of one full time staff member. It is important, then, that the occasion reflects both quality and effectiveness.[20] The information imparted at this time should be fundamental to the nursing activity which follows and consequently the care the patient receives throughout the span of her hospital stay. Nursing care often requires adjustment during a working shift as well as between one shift and another. It is therefore necessary for nurses to record and hand over information to other colleagues to promote quality and continuity of care and to allow forward planning.[20]

The transfer of a patient's care from one clinician to another is commonly referred to as the "handoff" and is an obvious example of a process which is prone to error and needing improvement. Inadequate communication can result in lost information, misinterpretation and misdirected or omitted actions. The scope of the issue is enormous. Handoffs occur between nurses, between physicians and between health providers at every level of the health care system. During the course of a patient's hospital stay, the number of communication handoffs is staggering. The patient usually presents to the labor and delivery unit (if she starts in the Emergency Department that is an additional opportunity in need of a handoff) and after delivery is transferred to the postpartum unit. It is not unusual for a laboring woman to see several shifts come and go, each bringing with them new providers who will need a report on the maternal-fetal status. She may also require visits to other departments during her stay. For example, she may require X-Rays or a return to the OR with a complication. Her baby or babies may require additional care in a transitional care unit or Neonatal Intensive Care Unit before being admitted to the normal newborn nursery. Each handoff represents a point of potential error or omission in communication.

The Joint Commission has included the improvement of communication among caregivers and the standardization of handoff communications as a National Patient Safety Goal (2E). The Joint Commission expects its accredited organizations to conduct patient handoffs as uninterrupted and interactive exchanges of relevant patient information with an opportunity for questions, allowing the oncoming caregiver to clarify any uncertainties that he or she may have. It is important to consider the relationship between written nursing reports and verbal handoffs: verbal handoffs should be used to supplement written reports, not to duplicate them.[21]

---

**Example of Lack of Information Given During a Handoff** [22]

A 27-year-old woman was admitted to the hospital at 42 weeks gestation for an induction of labor. The reason for induction was post dates and suspected fetal macrosomia. The patient received epidural anesthesia and was fully dilated 14 hours after admission. The station was 0-+1 with marked caput according to the nurse's notes. After pushing for 3 hours, the patient was noted to be exhausted with no progress made. A note written at 18:50 stated that the patient was prepped for delivery and a vacuum applied. The next note at 19:23 stated "VAVD of 9 pound 8 ounce viable girl. Apgars were 5 and 8 and report was given to the night nurse."

At 30 minutes of age, the nursery nurse reported that the baby's vital signs were: T-36.8 (skin to skin), P-168, R-70. Thirty minutes later they were charted as: T-35.9 (skin to skin), with 3 blankets and a hat. P-180, R-76.

The color was noted to be pale and the baby had fair tone. There was large caput with bruising and marked molding. The baby was placed under a warmer and a cephalhematoma was questioned. Twenty minutes later, the baby was apneic, cyanotic and bradycardic. Upon transfer to the NICU she was found to have massive bilateral intracranial hemorrhages.

During discovery, the parents testified that at least 12-13 separate traction efforts were made over a 30 minute period and they also heard "loud popping sounds." None of this was documented. The night nurse also testified that she was not aware that a vacuum had been used.

---

> This is clearly a case in which a proper "handoff" would have included information to the nursery nurse that a vacuum extractor had been used and that she needed to be aware of any signs of complications. Risk management in this case also included that nurses should receive appropriate education and training, be familiar with the policies and procedures and documentation guidelines regarding vaginal assisted vacuum deliveries.

The important components of a successful handoff include:[20, 23, 24]

- Conducting face-to-face oral updates with interactive questioning
- Sharing of experiences and expert knowledge of clinical situations
- Use of role playing to teach new nurses how to effectively communicate handoffs
- Delaying of transfer of care responsibility when there is concern about status of the process or the inability of the incoming provider to safely handle the situation
- Limiting interruptions and other activities
- Allowing both parties to initiate topics
- Allowing time for the receiver to review pertinent data before the handoff
- Presentation of the data in the same order every time
- The receiver reading back acquired information (ie. lab results, medication orders)
- Transferring responsibility unambiguously
- Assessment of patient status together at the bedside
- Development of protocols for what type of information must be included in a handoff for each clinical situation
- Regular observation of handoffs in progress to evaluate the process and develop ideas for improvement
- Education of student nurses so that they will be prepared for this important aspect of their working day

It is important to note that the hand-off process may vary depending on circumstances. For example, when a nurse is relieved for lunch or a break, information for the safe care of the patient must be conveyed so that missed information does not lead to a breach in the standard of care. While the report may not need to be extensive, the relieving nurse must have the information that is essential to rendering safe care.

**Take Home Message**

Be proactive in encouraging open interactions with your colleagues. Remember that accurate, effective, comprehensive and collegial communication during shift report promotes critical thinking which leads to the patient receiving an evidence based practice plan of care. This can only enhance safe care for mothers and babies.

## Maintaining Respectful Professional Interactions Is Essential to Teamwork and Patient Safety

Nurse-physician communication can be conflictive to the point of dysfunctional. This conflict arises from competition for status and power and different values and beliefs.[25] Anything that undermines open communication and effective interdisciplinary teamwork can pose a threat to patient safety. One such threat is disruptive or intimidating behavior demonstrated by professionals in the healthcare setting. The spectrum of this type of behavior includes angry outbursts, rudeness, verbal attacks, physical threats or aggressive physical contact, non compliance with existing policies, sexual harassment, idiosyncratic, inconsistent, or passive aggressive orders, derogatory comments about the organization, and disruption of the smooth functioning of the healthcare team.[26]

It must be remembered that each member of the team is essential in providing safe care to both mother and baby. Therefore, no one discipline is more important than another. However, disruptive behavior among nurses and physicians is not uncommon. Rosenstein and O'Daniel[27] reported results from a survey which was distributed to 50 VHA hospitals across the country. Results of 1,500 survey participants were evaluated and nurses were reported to have behaved disruptively almost as frequently as physicians. Most respondents perceived disruptive behavior as having negative or worsening effects on stress, frustration, concentration, communication, collaboration, information transfer, and workplace relationships. Even more disturbing were the respondents' perceptions of negative or worsening effects of disruptive behavior on adverse events, medical errors, patient safety, patient mortality, the quality of care, and patient satisfaction. Of survey respondents, 17% knew of an adverse event that occurred as a result of disruptive behavior; 78% of them thought the event could have been prevented.

**Examples of Respondent Comments from the Disruptive Behavior and Clinical Outcomes: Perceptions of Nurses and Physicians Survey**[27]

"There are several MDs on the staff who have rude and intimidating personalities. These physicians do not respect the nurses and make for a stressful environment."

"Disruptive behavior is not unique to physicians. Some nurses exhibit an air of superiority which makes communication difficult."

"Physicians who are disruptive are usually chronic disrupters and have run-ins with several nurses. There are also nurses who are chronic disrupters. These people are often avoided by other staff which leads to lowered communication. I am sure that a serious incident is just around the corner."

"The environment of hostility and disrespect is very distracting and causes minor errors. I have caught myself in the middle of mislabeling specimens after confrontations that have been upsetting."

"The communication between OB and delivery RN was hampered because of MD behavior. It resulted in a poor outcome in the newborn."

Disruptive or intimidating behavior can contribute to near misses and adverse outcomes directly by inhibiting communications between members of the health care team, decreasing the willingness to question and discuss orders or treatment plans, or by causing "work arounds" to avoid contact and discussions with disruptive practitioners.[26] Some nurses play the "nurse-doctor game" all too often and this is not only dysfunctional and dishonest but potentially dangerous.

**Did You Know?**
Effective January 1, 2009, the Joint Commission has a new Leadership standard (LD. 03.01.01) that addresses disruptive and inappropriate behaviors in two of its elements of performance:
EP 4: The hospital/organization has a code of conduct that defines acceptable and disruptive inappropriate behaviors.
EP 5: Leaders create and implement a process for managing disruptive and inappropriate behavior.

In addition, standards in the Medical Staff chapter have been organized to follow six core competencies to be addressed in the credentialing process, including interpersonal skills and professionalism.

Source: Behaviors that undermine a culture of safety. The Joint Commission Sentinel Event Alert #40, July 9, 2008.

---

**The following is an example from the American Association of Critical Care Nurses Standards for Establishing and Sustaining Healthy Work Environments (2005)**[28]

At 3:30 a.m. in a busy ICU, a nurse prepares to give insulin to a patient with an elevated blood sugar level. The sliding scale doses of insulin on the medication sheet are unclear and the physician's order sheet is difficult to read. From past experience, the nurse knows how late night calls to this physician often result in verbal outbursts and demeaning slurs, no matter how valid the inquiry.

Needing to act but not wanting another harassing encounter with the physician, she makes a judgment of the appropriate dose and administers the insulin. Two hours later, she finds the patient completely unresponsive. To treat the critically low blood sugar level, she administers concentrated injections of glucose and calls for additional help. Despite all attempts to restore the patient's brain to consciousness, he never awakens and his brain never functions normally again.

---

Verbal abuse prevents effective communication as well as being disrespectful. Teamwork cannot be successful if disruptive behavior is not addressed and allowed to continue. It is essential that health care organizations recognize the importance of addressing such issues and have a plan in place when such occurrences happen The following organizational processes for disruptive clinician behavior have been suggested:[29]

- A universal code of conduct should provide guidance to both clinicians and administrators.
- Expectations for professional behavior should be outlined explicitly in institutional policies for good citizenship and reaffirmed by both leaders and each clinician on an annual basis during contract renewal and performance reviews.
- Behavior should not be qualified by discipline (throwing instruments, "temper tantrums," or demeaning comments should not be tolerated by

any clinician). Exceptions should not be made because he or she is, "a good doctor or nurse otherwise," "we need their patient volume," or they are "one of the few who are always willing to work overtime."

- Processes for reporting disruptive behavior and behavior code enforcement should be widely disseminated and their use actively encouraged.
- There should be accountability and meaningful follow-up with clear actionable implications.
- Each instance should be addressed in a timely manner rather than delaying interventions until "trends" are apparent.

Johnson[30] suggests the following actions to stem disruptive behaviors in the moment:
- React immediately with the response that is appropriate to the situation, such as by saying, "I can't answer you while you are yelling," "If you lower your voice, I can respond" or "Your behavior is unacceptable for a professional."
- Redirect the focus onto the patient's needs to depersonalize the issue.
- Move the conflict away from patient care areas. If you fell threatened, move closer to other staff.
- If your unit has a signal when such behavior is occurring, use it so that you have witnesses. Witnesses serve the primary purpose of corroborating the events that have transpired, but some abusers also will modify their behavior if others are present.
- When a colleague provokes your anger, eschew retaliatory hostility by defusing the immediate anger you feel by using relaxation techniques.[31]
- After the anger subsides, plan to discuss the matter with the offender. It may help to practice your approach with a friend beforehand.[31]

It should also be noted that those caring for the patient should not be abused or intimidated by family members or visitors. People have been known to become very upset about anything from disagreeing with the patient's plan of care (the need for a cesarean section as opposed to a vaginal delivery) to room accommodations. Outbursts or rude, threatening behavior should never be tolerated as they are not only unfair and disrespectful to a team whose goal is to care for the patient and her baby, but can also sabotage the safe delivery of that care. The nursing supervisor and/or hospital security should be notified whenever inappropriate behavior presents itself.

**Figure 2-1** depicts the American Association of Critical Care Nurses[28] six standards and the interdependence of each standard to create a healthy work environment.

For example, effective decision making, appropriate staffing, meaningful recognition and authentic leadership depend upon skilled communication and true collaboration. Likewise, authentic leadership is imperative to ensure sustainable implementation of the other behavior-based standards. A healthy work environment further leads to clinical excellence and optimal patient outcomes.

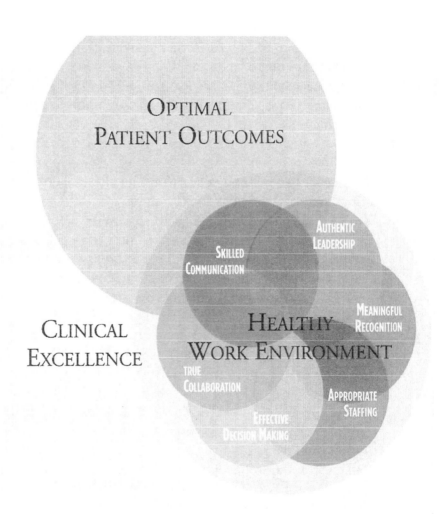

**Figure 2-1    Interdependence of Healthy Work Environment, Clinical Excellence and Optimal Patient Outcomes**

Reproduced with permission from: American Association of Critical Care Nurses (2005). <u>American Association of Critical Care Nurses Standards for Establishing and Sustaining Healthy Work Environment</u>. Author: California.

**Strategies Designed to Prevent Individual Error and Create a Culture of Safety**

- Leaders make sure that they are visibly committed to change and enable staff to openly share safety information
- Safe staffing patterns are maintained. (**see Table 2-2**)
- People are not merely encouraged to work toward change; they take action when it is needed
- Ensure complete orientations and be sure to stress the philosophy of your unit striving for high reliability and safety
- Make expectations of all staff members clear
- Manage workplace fatigue and stress: provide adequate staffing; breaks; reasonable work schedules - limit working different shifts in a short time span; support the overstressed employee with counseling and being sensitive to scheduling
- Decrease reliance on memory: use checklists; written, easily accessible protocols
- Decrease reliance on vigilance: constraints which do not allow fatal errors: free flow protection; bar coding
- Reduce or eliminate handoffs: staff scheduling
- Reduce the need for manual calculations: have calculators readily available; double check policy in place; preprinted laminated charts
- Design useful policies: reasonable, clear, concise
- Develop standardized unit practices based on evidence based practice: involve staff in reviewing and updating practices; encourage staff to join professional organizations such as the Association of Women's Health, Obstetric and Neonatal Nursing (AWHONN)
- Have accurate up-to-date information readily available: Unit policies on line; pharmacology text readily available or on line; create a library of current textbooks, standards and guidelines from professional associations; subscription to the Cochrane database of Systematic Reviews
- Incorporate the principles of team training into the everyday functioning of the unit
- Encourage patients to be actively involved in their care and treatment and to report any concerns they may have about the care they are or are not receiving
- Use errors as a learning experience
- Experts need to remember that novices require time to learn and need to be "nurtured" so that they too will become expert; taking the

time to explain things now will benefit everyone in the future
- Disruptive clinician behavior should not be tolerated and a system should be in place to address such behaviors

Adapted from: Nolan, TW (2000). Education and debate: System changes to improve patient safety. British Medical Journal, 320 (7237), 771-773; Simpson, K & Knox,G (2003). Adverse perinatal outcomes: Recognizing & preventing common accidents. AWHONN Lifelines,7 (3) 225-235.

**Table 2-2  Recommended Registered Nurse/Patient Ratios for Perinatal Care Services**

| Registered Nurse/Patient Ratio | Care Provided |
|---|---|
| Intrapartum | |
| 1:2 | Patients in labor |
| 1:1 | Patients in second stage of labor |
| 1:1 | Patients with medical or obstetrical complications |
| 1:2 | Oxytocin induction or augmentation of labor |
| 1:1 | Coverage for initiating epidural anesthesia |
| 1:1 | Circulation for Cesarean section |
| Antepartum/Postpartum | |
| 1:6 | Antepartum and postpartum patients without complications |
| 1:2 | Patients in postoperative recovery |
| 1:3 | Antepartum and postpartum patients with complications but in stable condition |
| 1:4 | Newborns and those requiring close observation |
| Newborns | |
| 1:6-8* | Newborns requiring only routine care |
| 1:3-4 | Normal mother-newborn couplet care |
| 1:3-4 | Newborns requiring continuing care |
| 1:2-3 | Newborns requiring intermediate care |
| 1:1-2 | Newborns requiring intensive care |
| 1:1 | Newborns requiring multi-system support |
| 1:1 or greater | Unstable newborns requiring complex critical care |

\*This ratio reflects traditional newborn nursery care. If breast feeding or couplet care is provided, a registered nurse coordinates and administers care for the mother and newborn couple (1:3-4 couples). If it is necessary to separate the well mother and newborn couple, and return the newborn to a central nursery, the mother-newborn registered nurse is still responsible for the mother-baby couple. Another registered nurse would provide care for the newborn in the central nursery. At least one registered nurse should be available at all times in each occupied basic care nursery when newborns are physically present in the nursery. Direct care of newborns in the nursery may be provided by ancillary personnel under the registered nurse's direct supervision. Adequate staff is needed to respond to acute and emergency situations at all times.

Used with permission of the American Academy of Pediatrics and the American College of Obstetricians and Gynecologists. Guidelines for Perinatal Care. 6th ed. 2007. Copyright held by AAP and ACOG.

**Importance of Measuring Culture**

To maximize the potential of patient safety initiatives, Smetzer[4] recommends regularly measuring culture at both the departmental and administrative level, identifying problem areas, sharing findings, and seeking feedback to motivate change. Measuring culture will help to establish a framework within which to justify change and demonstrate positive results. A minimal set of domains to be measured should include:[4]

> *Leadership.* Are board members, executives, managers and medical staff committed to patient safety?
> *Empowerment.* Are frontline caregivers empowered to "stop the line" or otherwise take action to put patient safety first?
> *Communication.* Is there an assumption of clinical competence in interactions between every doctor and every nurse? Ancillary staff?
> *Commitment.* Is patient safety just the "flavor of the month" or ingrained in your long-term strategic plan?
> *Teamwork.* Do care team members act as individual agents or embrace the concept of "we"?
> *Transparency.* Does a culture of secrecy prevail or one of transparency, where information is shared openly among clinicians and with patients and families?
> *Risk tolerance.* Do individuals engage in at-risk behavior based on habit or pressure, or are they coached to make safe behavioral choices every time once the system-based causes of the at-risk behavior are resolved?

> *Justice/accountability*. Does the organization encourage individual accountability by distinguishing between human error, at-risk behavior, and reckless actions?

---

**Take Home Message**

Knowledge, attitude and performance are seen as team-related outcomes and it is the interactions of leadership, situation monitoring, mutual support and communication with these outcomes that is the basis of a team striving to deliver safe, quality care.

---

**Obstetrical "Never Events"**

The importance of our maintaining a commitment to establishing and promoting a culture of safety is further strengthened when we look at the following list of events. In 2002, the National Quality Forum (NQF)[32] published a list of 27 adverse healthcare events that are serious and largely preventable. They have been deemed "Never Events". Simpson[33] has extended the list, adding situations which we need to strive to make sure never happen to our mothers and/or babies. The following are obstetrical "Never Events":

- ❖ Infant abduction
- ❖ Infant death or serious disability (kernicterus) associated with failure to identify and treat neonatal hyperbilirubinemia
- ❖ Infant discharged to the wrong person
- ❖ Maternal or infant death or serious disability associated with a hemolytic reaction resulting from the administration of ABO-incompatible blood or blood products
- ❖ Maternal death or serious disability associated with labor and birth in a low risk pregnancy while being cared for in a healthcare facility
- ❖ Maternal or infant death or serious disability associated with a medication error, e.g., errors associated with the 5 *rights* which includes overdose of Oxytocin, Misoprostol, and magnesium sulfate
- ❖ Wrong surgical procedure performed on a mother or infant (e.g. circumcision, tubal ligation)
- ❖ Retention of a foreign object in a mother or infant after surgery or another procedure
- > Maternal death after pulmonary embolism in untreated patient with known high risk factors for deep vein thrombosis
- > Infant breastfed by wrong mother or breast milk given to wrong infant
- > Death or serious disability of a fetus/infant with a reassuring fetal heart

> rate pattern or mother's admission for labor barring any acute unpredictable event
> Prolapsed cord after elective rupture of membranes with the fetus at high station
> Prolonged periods of untreated uterine hyperstimulation during Oxytocin or Misoprostol administration
> Prolonged periods of a non reassuring fetal heart rate pattern during labor unrecognized and/or untreated with the usual intrauterine resuscitation techniques
> Fundal pressure during birth involving shoulder dystocia
> Ruptured uterus following prostaglandin administration for cervical ripening/labor induction to a woman with a known uterine surgical scar
> Missed administration of RhoGAM to a mother who is an appropriate candidate
> Circumcision without pain relief measures
> Neonatal group B streptococcus or HIV infection after missed intrapartum chemoprophylaxis
> Infant death or disability after multiple attempts with multiple instruments to affect an operative vaginal birth
> Infant death or disability after prolonged periods of repetitive coached second-stage labor pushing efforts during a nonreassuring FHR pattern

> (Proposed by Kathleen Rice Simpson, PhD, RN, FAAN)

---

**Take Home Message**

Reducing the risk of liability exposure and avoiding preventable injuries to mothers and infants during labor and birth can be relatively easy when all members of the perinatal team (nurses, nurse midwives, and physicians) agree to follow two basic tenets of clinical practice: *use applicable evidence and/or published standards and guidelines as the foundation for care* and whenever a clinical choice is presented, *choose patient safety rather than production.*

Simpson & Knox. (2003). Common areas of litigation related to care during labor and birth: Recommendations to promote patient safety and decrease risk exposure. <u>Journal of Perinatal and Neonatal Nursing</u>, 17 (2), 110-125.

1. Boyer MM. Root cause analysis in perinatal care: Health care professionals creating safer health care systems. *J Perinat Neonat Nurs.* 2001; 15:40-54.

2. To err is human: Building a safer health system. Washington DC: National Academy of Science; 1999.

3. Maddox P, Wakefield M, Bull J. Patient safety and the need for professional and educational change. *Nursing Outlook.* 2001; 49:8-13.

4. Smetzer J, Navarra M. Measuring change: A key component of building a culture of safety. *Nursing Economics.* 2007; 25:49-51.

5. Institute of Medicine. Crossing the quality chasm: A new health system for the 21st century. Washington DC: National Academies Press; 2001.

6. Benner P, Sheets V, Uris P, Malloch K, Schwed K, Jamison D. Individual, practice, and system causes of errors in nursing: A taxonomy. *J Nurs Adm.* 2002; 32:509-523.

7. Reason JT. *Managing the Risks of Organizational Accidents.* Aldershof,UK: Ashgate; 1997.

8. Simpson KR, Knox GE. Adverse perinatal outcomes: Recognizing, understanding & preventing common accidents. *AWHONN Lifelines.* 2003; 7:225-235.

9. Miller LA. System errors in intrapartum electronic fetal monitoring: A case review. *J Midwifery Womens Health.* 2005; 50:507-516.

10. Mahlmeister LR. Legal issues and risk management. best practices in perinatal care: Reporting "near misses" and "good catches" as a risk reduction strategy. *J Perinat Neonat Nurs.* 2006; 20:197-199.

11. Reason J. Human error: Models and management. BMJ. 2000; 320:768-770.

12. Edwards WH. Patient safety in the neonatal intensive care unit. *Clinics in Perinatology,.* 2005; 32:97-106.

13. Leape LL. Reporting of adverse events. *N Engl J Med.* 2002; 347:1633-1638.

14. Kaushal R, Bates DW, Landrigan C, et al. Medication errors and adverse drug events in pediatric inpatients. *JAMA.* 2001; 285:2114-2120.

15. Salas E, Sims D, Klein C, Burke C. Can teamwork enhance patient safety?

Forum. 2003; 23:5-9.

16. Simpson K, Creehan P. *Perinatal Nursing*. 3rd ed. Philadelphia: Lippincott Williams & Wilkins:; 2008.

17. Miller LA. Safety promotion and error reduction in perinatal care: Lessons from industry. *J Perinat Neonat Nurs*. 2003; 17:128-138.

18. Mann S, Marcus R, Sach B. Lessons from the cockpit: How team training can reduce errors on L & D. *Contemporary OB/GYN*. 2006:1-7.

19. Groff H, Augello T. From theory to practice: An interview with Dr. Michael Leonard. *Forum*. 2003; 23:10-13.

20. Sherlock C. The patient handover: A study of its form, function and efficiency. *Nurs Stand*. 1995; 9:33-36.

21. Footitt B. Ready for report. *Nurs Stand*. 1997; 11:22-23.

22. Mahlmeister L. Legal issues and risk management. Best practices in perinatal and neonatal nursing: Cervical ripeners and the induction of labor. *J Perinat Neonat Nurs*. 2005; 19:97-99.

23. Wilkie A, Greenberg C. Communication handoffs:One hospital's approach. *Forum*. 2007; 25:10-11.

24. Simpson KR. Perinatal patient safety. Handling handoffs safely. *MCN*. 2005; 30:152.

25. Arford PH. Nurse-physician communication:An organizational accountability. *Nurs Econ*. 2005; 23: 72-77.

26. Veltman L. Disruptive behavior in obstetrics: A hidden threat to patient safety. *American Journal of Obstetrics and Gynecology*. 2007; 196:587.e1-587.e5.

27. Rosenstein A, O'Daniel M. Disruptive behavior & clinical outcomes: receptions of nurses and physicians. *American Journal of Nursing*. 2005; 105:55-64.

28. American Association of Critical Care Nurses, ed. AACN *Standards for Establishing and Susataining Healthy Work Environments*. California: AACN; 2005.

29. Simpson KR. Perinatal patient safety. disruptive clinician behavior. *MCN*. 2007; 32:64.

30. Johnson CL, Martin SL, Markle-Elder S. Stopping verbal abuse in the workplace. *Am J Nurs.* 2007; 107:32-34.

31. Thomas SP. Professional development. 'horizontal hostility': Nurses against themselves: How to resolve this threat to retention. *Am J Nurs.* 2003; 103:87-8, 91.

32. National Quality Forum. Serious reportable events in healthcare. Washington, DC: Author; 2002.

33. Simpson KR. Perinatal patient safety. Obstetrical "never events". *MCN.* 2006; 31:136.

# CHAPTER 3

# Common Alleged Deviations from the Standard of Nursing Care & Risk Management

*Claims of negligence related to the nurse's affirmative duty have grown over the years. The legal doctrine upholding the physician as "captain of the ship" has been considerably eroded.*

*Laura Mahlmeister[1]*

---

**Did You Know?**

Before 1950, nurses had only Florence Nightingale's early treatments, plus reports of court cases, to use as standards. In 1950, the American Nurses Association (ANA) published the "Code of Ethics for Nursing" which was a general mandate stating that nurses should offer nursing care without prejudice and in a confidential and safe manner. This code marked the beginning of written nursing standards. It was not until 1974 that maternal-child nursing, as a specialty, established distinct standards under ANA.

Source: Helm, A. (2003). <u>Nursing malpractice: Sidestepping legal minefields</u>. Philadelphia: Lippincott Williams & Wilkins. Pg. 125.

---

The following are often cited as deviations from the standard of care for perinatal nurses. **Table 3-1** includes additional noted deviations, allegations, standards and guidelines and recommendations.

**Failure to Recognize Maternal/Fetal Risk Pattern**

The identification of high-risk patients is often the responsibility of the nurse because the high-risk status often does not appear until the patient presents in labor. Allegations against nurses claim that they failed to know the patient's history and/or did not assess the patient on an ongoing basis so that risks were not identified.[2]

Today's obstetrical population has changed in that we are now seeing patients who in previous years would have been rare. Women are choosing to have babies at an advanced age. These patients have a longer medical history

# Common Alleged Deviations from the Standard of Nursing Care & Risk Management

**Table 3-1 Common Areas of Litigation, Allegations, Standards and Guidelines and Recommendations**

| Common Areas of Litigation | Common Allegations | Standards & Guidelines | Recommendations |
|---|---|---|---|
| Telephone Triage (calls made to the labor & delivery unit) | Failure to: <br> • Accurately assess maternal-fetal status over the phone <br> • Advise the woman to seek inpatient evaluation and treatment <br> • Correctly communicate maternal-fetal status to the primary care provider <br> Failure of the physician or midwife to come to the hospital to see the woman as requested. | The liability for assessing and diagnosing conditions of pregnancy and labor should remain with the primary care providers rather than assumed by the institution. | Telephone advice to pregnant women by labor and delivery nurses should be limited to two comments: *call* your primary care provider or *come* to the hospital. |
| Telephone Triage (Office based) | • Failure to diagnose <br> • Delay of treatment <br> • Improper treatment <br> • Failure to follow-up <br> • Poor telephone procedures <br> • Breech of confidentiality <br> • Inadequate documentation | Responsibilities of the registered nurse or CNM performing telephone triage include: <br> • Assess the severity and urgency of the problem as emergent, urgent or non-urgent. <br> • Implement the appropriate action <br> • Evaluate the patient's understanding of the instructions given. <br> • Document all aspects of the contact which may be in a log or the patient's chart. | Listen carefully to the caller, etc. Avoid jumping to conclusions or using medical jargon. Try to talk to the person directly and not go through a second party (i.e. husband, friend). Always use medically approved protocols which are reviewed and updated on a regular basis. Orient and train staff in telephone triage protocols, policies and procedures, phone encounter techniques, dealing with difficult calls, and documentation. Develop a schedule to conduct chart audits to evaluate consistency, accuracy and |

44

adherence to established protocols. Attend conferences, workshops, and continuing education offerings to establish competency in communication skills, assessment, and telephone triage.

Protocols must reflect that the:
- Advice given to the patient is accurate, complete and consistent.
- Time frame for the patient to reevaluate her condition is provided.
- Instructions given to the patient include her need to call back, go to the emergency room or go to the labor and delivery unit if her symptoms are not relieved in the designated time frame.

The triage nurse should:
- Always err on the side of caution by making an appointment for the patient or have them report to labor and delivery.
- Never refuse to make an appointment for the patient if the patient requests one.
- Consult with the physician while the patient remains on the phone if the nurse believes the protocol does not completely address the patient's situation.

# Common Alleged Deviations from the Standard of Nursing Care & Risk Management

| | | | |
|---|---|---|---|
| | • Emphasize to the patient that the patient is responsible for calling back or seeking further care if circumstances worsen or fail to improve. | | |
| Emergency Medical Treatment and active Labor Act (EMTALA) (EMTALA is triggered whenever any pregnant woman presents to a hospital and requests care.) | Three fundamental patient care obligations must be met under EMTALA 1. An adequate medical screening exam must be provided for all patients. 2. Stabilization treatment within the capabilities of the hospital is provided to every patient with an emergency medical condition. 3. Transfer/discharge is conducted according to EMTALA statute guidelines. | Failure to: • Comply with all components of EMTALA • Perform a medical screening exam • Provide a physician to assess maternal-fetal status Failure of a physician to come to the hospital to see the woman prior to discharge or transfer. Transfer or discharge of a woman in active labor or with an unstable medical complication of pregnancy. Transfer or discharge of a woman in active labor based on her inability to pay or lack of insurance. | Education of staff as to: 1. the nature and intent of the law 2. the forms that need to be filled out regarding physician authorization or certification for transfer, patient request for treatment or transfer, patient refusal for stabilization or transfer 3. signage requirement 4. record keeping (i.e. logs) Documentation of all education, consents, evaluation and transfer information before transferring to another institution or discharging home. |
| Informed Consent | The JCAHO standard for informed consent requires a mutual understanding between the patient and physician. The consent should be obtained by the person performing the procedure | Failure to: Obtain informed consent | Effective communication must be assured. Several things that can help address this are: 1. Use plain language and avoid complex medical terminology. 2. Have a medical interpreter available if necessary. |

| | | | |
|---|---|---|---|
| | | 3. Provide visual aids and illustrations.<br>4. Have the patient describe (*Teach Back*) what you have told her.<br>5. Document what has been told to the patient and their understanding.<br><br>**REMEMBER**: If there is any doubt that the patient has not received informed consent, the nurse has an obligation to contact the provider before the procedure commences. | Avoid:<br>• fundal pressure to shorten an otherwise normal second stage of labor<br>• fundal pressure during shoulder dystocia<br>• clinical<br>• disagreements about fundal pressures at the bedside in front of the patient by having an agreed upon policy.<br>Refer to clinical risk management guidelines for fundal pressure (provided by professional liability insurance carriers) when developing unit guidelines. |
| Fundal Pressure During the Second Stage of Labor | Application of fundal pressure:<br>• during the second stage of labor resulting in shoulder dystocia and/or other maternal-fetal injuries<br>• during shoulder dystocia further impacting the shoulder, delaying birth resulting in fetal injuries | Fundal pressure during the second stage of labor is associated with risks of adverse outcomes to:<br>Mother<br>• perineal injuries: sphincter tears; uterine rupture and inversion; pain; hypotension; respiratory distress; abdominal bruising; fractured ribs; liver rupture<br>Infant<br>• Brachial plexus injuries; fracture of the humerus and clavicle; hypoxia; asphyxia; death; increased intracranial pressure; umbilical cord compression; subgaleal | |

| | | | Read: Mayberry, L. et al (2000). *Second Stage Labor Management: Promotion of Evidence-Based Practice and a Collaborative Approach to Patient Care.* AWHONN. |
|---|---|---|---|
| Forceps and Vacuum-Assisted Birth (Operative Birth) | Application of forceps/vacuum at high station resulting in maternal-fetal injury. Inappropriate timing or application of forceps resulting in fetal injuries. Excessive time of vacuum application.<br>Use of:<br>• Excessive force<br>• Vacuum for rotation of the fetal head<br>• Excessive pressures during vacuum-assisted birth | hemorrhage; spinal cord injuries<br><br>Only those individuals with privileges to perform an operative birth are to carry them out. Personnel must be readily available to perform a cesarean section should the operative birth be unsuccessful. Indications for application of forceps or vacuum (only after the fetal head has been determined to be engaged and the cervix is fully dilated) include:<br>• Nulliparous women: prolonged second stage with no progress in 3 hours with regional anesthesia or 2 hours without regional anesthesia.<br>• Multiparous women: lack of continued progress for 2 hours with regional anesthesia or 1 hour without anesthesia.<br>• Suspicion of immediate or potential fetal compromise.<br>• Shortening of the second. | Education of staff should include:<br>• The risks of forceps/vacuum delivery to both mother and baby.<br>• Responsibilities in assisting the provider with an operative delivery.<br>• Importance of monitoring the fetal heart during the procedure. Importance of supporting the woman through the procedure.<br>• Signs and symptoms of complications of an operative delivery to both mother and baby.<br>• Documentation of the procedure used and initial newborn assessment.<br>• Importance of notifying clinicians caring for the newborn that a vacuum device was used so that they can adequately monitor the newborn for signs and |

48

| | |
|---|---|
| symptoms of device related injuries (i.e. subgaleal hematoma).<br><br>A unit policy which addresses the use of vacuum devices and forceps should be in place.<br><br>Read:<br>Food and Drug Administration (1998). *Need for caution when using vacuum assisted devices* (Public Health Advisory). Washington, DC: Author. | stage for maternal benefit<br>Forceps:<br>• Adhere to ACOG criteria for types of forceps births<br>- outlet, low and mid.<br>High forceps should not be permitted or attempted.<br>Vacuum-assisted vaginal birth:<br>• Follow the manufacturer's guidelines for the vacuum device being used.<br>• The vacuum pressure should not exceed 500-600 mm Hg and should be released as soon as the contraction ends and the patient stops pushing. Progress should be seen with each traction attempt and the procedure abandoned after 3 pulls. Traction should only be applied while the woman is actively pushing.<br>• Timing of the vacuum procedure begins from the moment of insertion of the cup into the vagina and should not be on the fetal head for longer than 20-30 minutes with the maximum pressure force not exceeding 10 minutes. |

# Common Alleged Deviations from the Standard of Nursing Care & Risk Management

|  |  |  |  |
|---|---|---|---|
|  |  | Only steady traction in the line of the birth canal should be used and rocking movements should never be applied to the device. The procedure should be abandoned if any of the following occur: • 2-3 pop-offs (check manufacturer's instructions) • evidence of scalp trauma • no descent with appropriate application and traction. | Plan in advance to have: • ultrasound equipment immediately available in the labor room to determine fetal presentation during the second stage of labor. • policies and procedures readily available for staff. • appropriate number of staff scheduled for labor, delivery and nursery. |
| Multiple Gestation | Failure to: • transfer care of high risk pregnancy to appropriate healthcare provider • diagnose multiple gestation • determine chorionicity of multiple gestation • accurately monitor all fetuses during labor and birth • have in place appropriate personnel and equipment during birth | Counseling which includes: • nutritional considerations • genetic • risks associated with multiple gestation for both mother and fetuses Determination of chorionicity. Delivery by 40 weeks. Confirmation of fetal number and presentations by ultrasound when labor is suspected. Continuous fetal monitoring of each fetus during labor. Each umbilical cord should be identified according to hospital policy so that cord blood specimens may be labeled correctly. |  |

| | | | |
|---|---|---|---|
| | | Appropriate, experienced pediatric, anesthesia and nursing staff should be notified and available at the delivery. | In cases where the mother:<br>1. Was treated for clinically suspected chorioamnionitis or the infant has signs of sepsis, a full workup is recommended regardless of gestational age or duration of maternal antibiotic therapy.<br>2. Was treated with antibiotics during labor based on the recommendations and the infant is under 35 weeks gestation or the mother received less than 4 hours of intrapartum antibiotic prophylaxis, limited observation for at least 48 hours is recommended with full diagnostic evaluation for the development of sepsis. |
| Prevention of Perinatal Group B Streptococcal Disease | Failure to adhere to the Centers for Disease Control and Prevention (CDC) guidelines for Group B Streptococcal (GBS) prophylaxis, resulting in neonatal infection and subsequent neonatal neurological damage and death. | All pregnant women should be screened at 35-37 weeks gestation for vaginal and rectal GBS colonization. Chemoprophylaxis should be given to:<br>• all pregnant women who present in labor or rupture membranes who have been identified as GBS carriers<br>• all pregnant women with GBS isolated from urine in any concentration during their current pregnancy<br>• all women with a history of having given birth to an infant with invasive GBS | |
| 30-Minute "Rule" | Failure to initiate a cesarean birth within 30 minutes of the decision to do so. | All hospitals offering labor and delivery services should be equipped to perform emergency cesarean delivery within 30 minutes of the decision to do so. The in-house anesthesia and pediatric staff responsible for | A plan should be in place so that all essential personnel are available to commence a cesarean section within a 30-minute time frame. Patients should be made aware during the antepartal period of the hospital's resources to be able to |

# Common Alleged Deviations from the Standard of Nursing Care & Risk Management

| | | | |
|---|---|---|---|
| Vaginal Birth After Cesarean Section (VBAC) | Failure to:<br>• Fully inform women with a history of a prior cesarean section or uterine scar of risks and benefits of a trial of labor for VBAC.<br>• Recognize signs and symptoms of uterine rupture. | covering the labor and delivery unit should be informed in advance when a complicated delivery is anticipated and when a patient with risk factors requiring a high acuity level of care is admitted.<br><br>Adhere to ACOG recommendations for appropriate candidates.<br>Avoid:<br>• Use of prostaglandin agents for cervical ripening and labor induction<br>• Excessive use of Oxytocin | perform emergency surgery so that they can decide whether or not to deliver at the institution. It should be kept in mind that some emergencies may not end in a positive outcome even if performed within the 30 minute time frame (i.e. prolapsed umbilical cord, abruption placenta, maternal cardiac arrest). Emergency drills for an emergency cesarean section are helpful in keeping staff competent and confident. Planning staffing needs accordingly ( i.e. is a scrub nurse or technician available on every shift?). The prudent nurse clarifies the emergent or non-emergent nature of the Cesarean section with the physician and documents the plan and time in the patient record. Staff education should include:<br>• The physiological and pharmacokinetic principles of cervical ripeners and oxytocin.<br>• Signs and symptoms of uterine rupture.<br>• Emergency measures in the event of a uterine rupture. |

| | | | |
|---|---|---|---|
| | • Treat uterine rupture in a timely manner.<br>• Have appropriate personnel and equipment during trial of labor for VBAC.<br>Use of:<br>• Excessive doses of Oxytocin during labor induction or augmentation resulting in uterine rupture.<br>• Prostaglandin agents for cervical ripening or labor induction for a woman with a history of a prior cesarean birth or uterine scar resulting in uterine rupture. | and hyperstimulation<br>Ensure that a full surgical and neonatal resuscitation team is in-house during the trial of labor. | Practice drills in the event of a uterine rupture. |
| Neonatal Hypoglycemia | Failure to:<br>• Monitor for hypoglycemia in the high risk neonate<br>• Recognize the signs of hypoglycemia | All infants at risk must be screened even if asymptomatic. Institutional policies for screening must be followed and results reported to the provider in a rapid fashion. | Education of perinatal nurses as to maternal and fetal risk factors.<br>All nurses should be aware of the hospital's policy for screening neonates. |

Adapted from: Simpson & Knox (2003). Common areas of litigation related to care during labor and birth. Recommendations to promote patient safety and decrease risk exposure. Journal of Perinatal and Neonatal Nursing. 17 (2). 110-125.; Dunn, P. Gies, M. & Peters, M. (2005). Perinatal litigation and related nursing issues. Clinics in Perinatology. 32 (1), 277-290.

and may have already acquired some of the illnesses seen as people age. Obesity is now of epidemic proportions and is fraught with potential complications such as diabetes, increased risk of intrauterine fetal demise, preeclampsia, shoulder dystocia and surgical complications, to name just a few. Women who suffer from some chronic illnesses are also now living to reproductive age. An example of this would be those with cystic fibrosis. Perinatal nurses are vulnerable to litigation should complications occur and this includes recognition of the symptoms of complications in the mother, fetus and neonate, resuscitation, and activation of emergency interventions.[3]

**Failure to Assess and Intervene**

Failure to perform a proper patient assessment is a common allegation in professional negligence cases. An assessment is the continuous collection of data used to identify a patient's actual and potential health needs.[2 P-88] Claims have been made that if a nurse properly assesses a patient on admission, a high risk status may be identified and an indication for transfer to a hospital that can provide a higher level of care may be recognized.[3] To avoid errors, an assessment should include the following:[4 P-237]

> ➤ the patient's chief complaint, preferably using direct quotes
> ➤ the primary nursing diagnosis (the most pressing problem or concern of the patient)
> ➤ the patient's history
> ➤ medication allergies
> ➤ physical assessment
> ➤ assessment of fetal well-being
> ➤ emotional status
> ➤ the patient's assessment of current pain level
> ➤ relevant psychosocial data
> ➤ analysis of the data collected[2 P-91]

The following are three examples of a nurse's failure to assess a patient.

---

**Failure to Properly Assess a Patient**

# 1  Mrs. G. G1 P0 at term arrived in labor and delivery on a very busy night. All of the rooms were occupied, so she had to wait to be put into a room. The patient was alert and oriented, and complaining of constant uterine pain. The admission note indicated that the fetus was tachycardic at 170 bpm, and that no regular uterine contractions were palpated. The patient reported leaking watery, bloody fluid and feeling decreased fetal movement for 8-10 hours. Forty-five minutes after her arrival, she was placed in a labor room. After 15 minutes, the electronic fetal monitor was

---

applied by a scrub technician. The RN entered the labor room 15 minutes later and noticed that the FHR was down to 60-70 bpm and had been for the previous 10 minutes. An emergency cesarean birth was performed, and an abruption of the placenta was found. The baby had Apgar scores of 0 and 3 and suffered profound neurologic damage. A lawsuit was filed against the hospital.

The nurse testified at her deposition that she suspected that the patient's placenta was abrupting, but she was busy with a second patient in active labor and was trying to get a third patient discharged so she could get the patient in question a bed. The nurse was found negligent for her failure to notify the nurse manager and ask for immediate help assessing the patient with a possible placental abruption.

### # 2  Wheeler v. Yettie Kersting Memorial Hospital (1993)

Mrs. Wheeler was taken to a small, community hospital in Texas for evaluation prior to transfer to a facility in Galveston. Nursing assessment at the small hospital revealed that the patient was 4 cm dilated, 70% effaced, and had bulging membranes. There was no mention in the medical record of the presenting part. Fetal monitoring and labor assessment were not performed. The nurses obtained permission from the physician on call at the hospital and a Galveston physician to transport Mrs. Wheeler. En route, Mrs. Wheeler's membranes ruptured and she proceeded to deliver the lower extremities and body of a breech infant. Head entrapment occurred and the fetus subsequently expired prior to complete delivery. The Texas Court of Appeals found the nurses responsible, in part, for their failure to completely assess the patient's condition and fetal presentation.

# 3  A one-day-old boy was transferred from a community hospital to a larger city hospital to rule out a GI bleed. He was receiving an infusion of calcium gluconate through an I.V. line in his right foot. On the third day, a nurse noted discoloration and edema at the IV site. As the baby was being transferred to another unit, a transfer note indicated the time the infiltration was discovered and the fact that the nurse checked the area before the transfer; however, these details do not appear in the medical record. In the medical record were flow sheets on which some of the original writing was scratched out and written over. When the baby's parents arrived and asked the staff about the injury, they were told that it was a blister. In addition, they were told by one of the physicians that the IV med was very caustic and was usually given to babies with heart problems. The parents had not been told that their baby had a heart problem and, in fact, did not.

## Common Alleged Deviations from the Standard of Nursing Care & Risk Management

The family brought suit against the nurse who cared for the baby when the infiltration occurred. Their allegations included failure to monitor the IV resulting in considerable scarring and subsequent loss of motion as the child grew.[5]

Helm[2] suggests that you keep the following legal issues in mind when assessing your patients:
> Have you entered into a nurse-patient relationship?
> Is your assessment continual?
> Have you communicated your assessment findings to the appropriate personnel and documented accordingly?
> Have you implemented the appropriate nursing orders?
> Have you identified the appropriate nursing diagnoses?
> Are you continuing to assess and reassess your patient throughout your shift especially after medication is administered or a procedure is done?

Rostant and Cady[4] make the following recommendations to avoid intervention errors:
> Record physician orders upon receiving them (READ BACK, if verbal)
> Confirm any orders that are illegible
> Respond to the physiology creating the fetal monitor tracing
> Interpret and react to clinical symptoms
> Carry out appropriate physician orders
> Use the five rights when administering medication
> Utilize good communication when conveying the medical condition of the patient
> Record both the communication and the response of the physician to status reports
> Initiate the Chain of Command when necessary

**Take Home Message**
Changes in the health status of a patient can be gradual or sudden and nurses are usually the first to see the changes and to take action. A nurse's accuracy in assessing and monitoring and her timely reporting of changes in health status to a physician can often mean the difference between life and death. The perinatal nurse's role is further complicated in that she always has at least two patients' welfare to consider.
Be certain that you are aware of your hospital's policies and national standards concerning the frequency of patient assessments (including vital

signs) and documentation. Do not dismiss these aspects of patient care because the patient appears well and stable.

### Failure to Recognize a Nonreassuring Fetal Heart Pattern

It is well recognized that electronic fetal monitoring by itself is ineffective in avoiding preventable adverse outcomes. It is effective only when used in accordance with published standards and guidelines by professionals skilled in correct interpretation and when appropriate timely intervention is based on that interpretation. Despite overwhelming evidence, any nonreassuring FHR pattern may be associated with subsequent newborn or childhood neurologic injury in the minds of parents and plaintiff attorneys.[6] The most common allegation is that the nurse did not interpret the electronic monitor tracing correctly. During discovery, the plaintiff's attorney will be sure to request that the fetal monitor strips be included with the woman's medical records. Electronic fetal monitoring is further discussed in Chapter 5.

**Figure 3-1** is a copy of the fetal monitoring tracing of a patient who presented at 33 4/7 weeks with a history of feeling no fetal movement for 2 days. Upon arrival, the patient was not placed on the fetal monitor because her two small children had accompanied her and the nurse told the physician that no one was available to watch the children. The physician's instructions were that the monitoring could wait. One hour later, the patient was put on the monitor and the strip was as depicted. A biophysical profile revealed a 2/10 with 2 points for amniotic fluid. Another hour later, a stat cesarean section was called and the baby delivered 50 minutes after that. Apgars were 1/2/4 and 7 at fifteen minutes. Cord pH was 7.09 and the baby's hemaglobin was 2.2. Neither the doctor nor the nurse recognized the pattern as being sinusoidal.

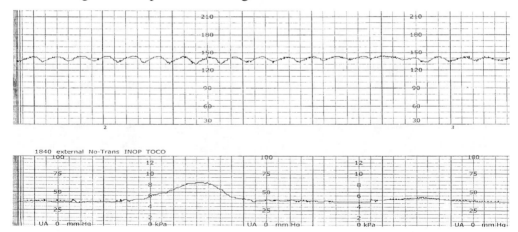

**Figure 3-1 Sinusoidal Pattern**

Common Alleged Deviations from the Standard of Nursing Care & Risk Management

**Failure to Appreciate a Deteriorating Fetal Condition**

It is essential that nurses are aware of changes that may occur over time. A fetus may start out displaying all the characteristics of a healthy fetus, but changes can and do occur during the stress of labor. Nurses must be vigilant of those changes.

---

**Example of Failure to Appreciate a Deteriorating Fetal Condition**

Ms. C. an 18-year-old primip was admitted to the hospital at 6 a.m. Oxytocin augmentation was started at noon. Although the fetal heart rate was initially normal, at 6 p.m. a prolonged deceleration to 60 bpm occurred and lasted 8 minutes. The physician was in attendance at this time. Subsequently, repeated severe variable and late decelerations were observed over the next 2 hours. The patient was taken to the delivery room at 8 p.m. Fetal heart rate monitoring was not conducted for the 22 minutes preceding the vaginal birth because a monitor was not available in the delivery room. The infant had an initial Apgar of 0 and required CPR by the respiratory therapist and nurses in the delivery room. A neonatologist did not examine the infant until 9 p.m.

Complaints against the nurse included failure to: recognize fetal distress; take action that would have led to a cesarean birth; assess the FHR in the delivery room which would have shown terminal bradycardia and failure to promptly call the neonatologist, which resulted in delayed treatment of the infant's acidosis.

Before trial the M.D. settled for $1 million and after the hospital went to trial, they were instructed to pay the plaintiff $10 million.

---

**Failure to Initiate and Sustain Intrauterine Resuscitation**

In response to nonreassuring signs, intrauterine resuscitative measures must be carried out. The main goal is to provide oxygen to the fetus. Intrauterine measures include: changing the patient's position, increasing intravenous fluids, administering oxygen at 8-10 liters via non-rebreather mask, discontinuing Oxytocin and notification of the provider. A tocolytic may also be ordered. All of these measures need to be documented in the patient's record whenever they are carried out.

---

**Example of Failure to Initiate and Sustain Intrauterine Resuscitation**
**Baptist Medical Center Montclair v. Wilson (1993)**

The patient, a VBAC candidate, was admitted to the labor and delivery unit in early labor. Hours later the patient experienced a sharp pain in her abdomen. Within moments the patient and her husband

---

noticed vaginal bleeding. The patient told the nurse she felt as though her stomach had ripped open and the baby had moved up toward the ceiling. Approximately 20 minutes later, the nurse performed a cervical exam and determined the patient's cervix was completely dilated. The fetal heart had dropped to 60 beats per minute. The nurse then notified the physician of her assessment, but did not report the sharp abdominal pain. Fifteen minutes later the physician examined the patient and found she was not dilated. An emergency cesarean section delivery followed. The delivery occurred almost one hour following the patient's report of abdominal pain. The patient had suffered a uterine rupture. Fetal distress resulted as the baby was pushed into the abdominal cavity causing placental abruption. The infant died at 5 months of age.

<u>Deviations from the Standard of Care That Were Noted at Trial</u>
Failure To:
Properly and completely assess the patient
Notify the physician of the sharp abdominal pain
Carry out intrauterine resuscitative measures

**Failure to Communicate with the Provider**

The nursing standard of care includes implementation of the nursing process in the provision of care to all patients. Communication processes among health care professionals and patients are an internal function in the performance of the standard of care provided to the patient. Failure to properly communicate or to notify the physician of significant findings is a frequent allegation against nurses.[4] Reviews of perinatal care (from individual cases and claims analysis) show that poor communication among providers and with patients contributes to care that is less than optimal and may increase the risk of malpractice claim. In one study of closed claims in obstetrics and gynecology, more than one-third of adverse events were associated with communication problems ranging from basic miscommunication among providers, to misunderstanding because of lack of common terminology, to delays in communication, and to total absence of communication.[7]

Communication problems often stem from several reasons including fear or intimidation, wanting to be "nice" to the physician and not "bother" him/her, failing to document conversations and not pursuing a provider who does not respond to the nurse's call. The nurse needs to stay focused on the needs of the patient and continue to realize that information must be communicated to the provider so that an appropriate plan of care can be initiated. It must also be remembered that nurses are now more specialized and the level of knowledge that the nurse is required to attain is significantly higher compared to the past.

# Common Alleged Deviations from the Standard of Nursing Care & Risk Management

Along with this increased knowledge, nurses have the responsibility and are expected to recognize and communicate any untoward findings.

---

**Examples of Poor Communication**

#1 A 32-year-old patient in her third trimester called her obstetrician's office complaining of a possible "strep throat" and relayed symptoms of a sore throat, swollen glands and a low grade fever. The office LPN did not consult the physician and gave the woman instructions to gargle with salt water and to take an over-the counter medication. After six days the patient called back and again talked with the office nurse complaining of no relief of symptoms. The nurse told the patient that she would be evaluated at her next appointment which was in 5 days. The next day the patient called back stating that she was now vomiting. Three hours later the patient called again, and the nurse consulted the physician who ordered Phenergan suppositories by telephone.

After continued vomiting and spotting, the patient came in to be evaluated by the physician who diagnosed "gastroenteritis" and admitted her to the hospital for hydration. The patient died within 6 hours after admission, with a diagnosis of group B streptococcus pyogenes.

The nurse was held liable for not communicating pertinent clinical information to the physician and the case settled for $750,000.

#2 **Goff v Physicians General Hospital of San Jose (1958)**

After delivery of the patient and making an incision into the patient's cervix to "relieve" a constrictive band of muscle, the physician inserted pelvic packing into the woman to control bleeding. He did not suture the incision. The patient was returned to her room and was being cared for by the nurse who attended the birth. When the nurse reported to the physician that she felt that the patient "was bleeding too much," he instructed her to observe the time it took for the perineal pads to become soaked.

The first time that the nurse checked the pads, she found "some" blood. Thirty minutes later, the pads were "approaching saturation". Fifteen minutes later, the pads were soaked and the nurse changed them. During her care, she did not take the patient's blood pressure, temperature, pulse or respiratory rate. The physician was not notified as the nurse was of the opinion that he would not "have come anyway."

At the end of the nurse's shift, the night nurse assessed the patient to be pulseless, cold and clammy, and "going into shock." The night nurse called the physician who arrived in 10 minutes, took the patient to the delivery room where she received oxygen and adrenalin. Due to inability

---

to access a vein, a blood transfusion was not started and the patient died of hemorrhage due to a lacerated cervix. The delivery nurse testified that she believed that an emergency existed when the pads had approached saturation and that the patient was in serious condition when the pads were soaked. The court concluded that the nurse's negligence in failing to properly assess the patient and communicate her findings to the physician contributed to her death.

Oftentimes, in charting, significant communications may be omitted from the document. Unfortunately, if the case progresses to litigation, the pertinent conversations cannot be remembered, much less reproduced as late entries.[4] By being cognizant of the need to document all significant communications the *he said/she said* scenario can also be avoided.

**Risk Management Strategies - Example of Effective Communication Techniques**
- Speak clearly using a congenial tone.
- Always act professional.
- Present facts in a methodical or chronological style.
- Use standardized medical terminology. (ie., NICHD terminology for EFM).
- Ask for clarification of orders - READ BACK.
- Communicate all relevant facts, abnormal findings and specific concerns.
- State your reasons if you do not agree with the plan.
- Be assertive and clear if the patient needs to be seen immediately.
- Inform the provider if you plan to initiate the chain of command.
- Document your conversation and the provider's response.

Adapted from: Rostant, D and Cady, R(1999). Liability issues in perinatal nursing. Lippincott: Philadelphia.

**Failure to Advocate for the Patient**
Modern law acknowledges the role of the nurse as a patient advocate. Nurses caring for mothers and newborns are highly educated individuals who have the responsibility to see that no harm comes to those in their care. A nurse who finds that a patient's safety and clinical outcome is at risk should initiate the chain of command communication process *before* there is irreversible damage.[4] While this requires strong communication skills and assertiveness, the nurse is obligated to use all resources that are available to her to protect and advocate for her patient.

## Common Alleged Deviations from the Standard of Nursing Care & Risk Management

Some members of the healthcare profession may still view nurses as those who perform tasks while caring for patients. The 1970s saw nursing evolving into a profession requiring critical thinking and knowledge rather than tasks and skills. The traditional model - nurses only following orders in a deferential relationship with physicians - has long since been replaced in most contemporary organizations and in most nurse-physician relationships.[8] It is difficult to believe that in this day and age, some physicians may not be aware that nurses have a legal and professional obligation to discuss potential problems and question a plan of care if necessary. This is a great opportunity to educate them to the fact that, by advocating for your patient, you are not only protecting the patient and yourself but also the hospital and physician from a potential lawsuit.

Thus, moral agency can be considered lacking when the nurse does not advocate for the best interests of the patient/family. When the nurse fails to question an inappropriate physician order, or fails to call a physician for a patient whose vital signs or lab reports are critical, or fails to heed patient or family requests for assistance, the lack of fiduciary concern and moral agency on behalf of patients causes harm and may be considered a source of substandard or erroneous nursing practice.[9]

It must be remembered that, although we are obligated to question a physician's potentially harmful or inappropriate order, you have no right to countermand by altering an order. Altering an order is a violation of the nurse practice act and exposes you to charges of insubordination and practicing medicine without a license.[10] This is another reason why the chain of command is so important.

**Failure to Initiate the Chain of Command**

The chain of command is a specific course of action that involves administrative and clinical lines of authority. **Figure 3-2** is one example of a chain of command algorithm. With a well-defined chain of command, a nurse who is presented with a challenging situation and is unable to resolve it herself can present the issue to successively higher levels of authority until a satisfactory resolution is reached. The nurse has an affirmative duty to call it to the attention of others who have the power and responsibility to evaluate and allay the nurse's concern, that is, to use the hospital's chain of command when any action by any person, in the nurse's opinion, is counter to good medical practice or they believe an intervention needed to protect the health or well-being of their patient is delayed by another practitioner's unwillingness or failure to act.[4, 11] Once the chain of command is activated, failure to continue until the issue of concern is appropriately resolved jeopardizes the patient's safety and the clinical team's liability. Bottom line, you do not have a choice. The chain of command is your obligation, Even if it turns out that you are not right in your assessment of the situation, that is okay and just move on. This is one time that is better to be safe than sorry and go with your instinct.

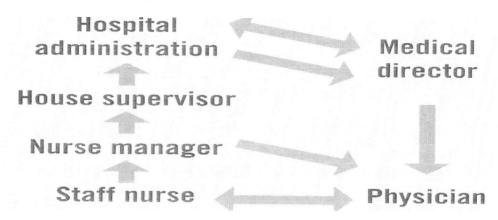

**Figure 3-2     Example of Chain of Command to Resolve Conflict**

Reproduced with permission from the Association of Women's Health, Obstetric and Neonatal Nurses. Fetal Heart Monitoring Principles and Practices. 3rd Ed. 2005. Kendall-Hunt Publishing: Iowa.

Nurses need to be cognizant of the value inherent in implementing a chain of command policy because they are frequently in the position to notice changes in patients that could necessitate altering the physician's orders or treatment plan.[12] All institutions should have a policy in place and make the chain of command readily available to their staff. Staff should also be assured that no punitive action will be taken should the chain of command be initiated. In a healthy clinical environment seeking clarification or confirmation should be encouraged and expected. Often a fresh perspective will offer ability to resolve the disagreement successfully and quickly for the patient and the providers involved.[13]

Nurses are often hesitant to document a physician's lack of response or a conflict which required the chain of command be initiated. It is clearly a very uncomfortable situation to be in, but should a malpractice suit occur and there is no documentation of the conversation between the nurse and provider, the nurse may be called upon to explain why she did not notify the physician. If there is no documentation, an opposing attorney will try to convince the jury that the conversation did not take place or the physician may forget that the nurse ever called. [4 P 115]

**Example of Documentation of the Chain of Command**

**Scenario**

      6 p.m. An 18-year-old G1 P0 presents to Labor and Delivery with a blood pressure of 160/110 and complaints of epigastric pain. She is 32 weeks pregnant. She tells you that she had pizza for dinner. You call the M.D. who is having dinner with his wife in a restaurant. He gives you an order for Maalox and tells you that he will not be in for at least 2 hours as they are celebrating his wife's birthday. You give the patient the Maalox and recheck her blood pressure 30 minutes later. Her B/P is now 164/114 and she is experiencing a headache. Reflexes are +3 with 2 beats of clonus. Her urine tests positive for a large amount of protein. You call the M.D. again and he tells you that you need to give the Maalox time to work. You are very concerned about the patient.

**Suggested Communication (SBAR) and Documentation**
**(6:30 p.m. 30 minutes after initial call)**
(Situation)
"Dr. Smith, I am calling you because I am very concerned about my patient who now has a blood pressure of 164/114, +3 reflexes with 2 beats clonus. Since we last spoke, she has developed a headache and protein in her urine"
(Background)
"This is an 18 year old primip who presented 30 minutes ago with a blood pressure of 160/110 and it is now 164/114."
(Assessment)
"I believe that she has preeclampsia which is worsening."
(Recommendation)
"Dr. Smith, it is my recommendation that a full set of preeclampsia labs needs to be drawn, an intravenous started and I am also requesting that you come to the hospital and see the patient immediately."

      Dr. Smith tells you to draw and send the labs, start an intravenous of Lactated Ringer's and that he will be finishing dinner within the hour. There is no need for him to come to the hospital as he will need the lab results in order to treat the patient.

**Suggested Communication (SBAR) and Documentation to his Response**

(Situation)

"Dr. Smith, I am very worried about this patient and would not be calling you if I did not think that the patient needed to be seen immediately."

(Background)

"Her blood pressure has increased in the past 30 minutes, she now has clonus and a headache."

(Assessment)

"Dr. Smith, I am concerned that this patient is becoming sicker."

(Recommendation)

"Dr. Smith, I am requesting for the second time that you come to the hospital and see your patient. She needs to be evaluated by a physician. If you are still not in agreement with my plan of care, I will plan to notify the charge nurse (and nursing supervisor if this is not resolved) as to my concerns and the seriousness of this matter."

Remember to document exactly what you told him and do not hesitate to be clear in documenting your recommendation. Suggestion:

*6:30 p.m. Dr. Smith notified of patient's increasing blood pressure, reflexes, headache and proteinuria. Apprised of my concern for patient and second request made that he come to the hospital to evaluate the patient. Dr. Smith verbalized that he would not be coming to the hospital at this time. Orders obtained for IV and labs. Dr. Smith made aware that I would be notifying the charge nurse (Susan James, RNC) per hospital Chain of Command Policy of my request that his patient be seen immediately. Will also plan to notify the nursing supervisor if unable to agree on a plan of care.*

Chain of command should not be the routine method of conflict resolution. Clinical disagreements that result in going up the chain of command can be detrimental to nurse-physician relationships. Soon after a clinical disagreement that results in use of the chain of command, all those involved should meet and calmly discuss what happened and why. Having an objective third party such as the risk manager present during this discussion may facilitate the interaction. Prospective plans should then be developed to avoid the situation in the future.[14] By addressing interpersonal conflicts early on, the consequences of letting them escalate into an area of potential liability can be averted.

**Did You Know?**

The results of a 2005 study entitled *Silence Kills*, discovered that 85% to 95% of the 1700 respondents (nurse, physicians, and administrators) were unable to speak up when observing colleagues act incompetently, break rules, and make mistakes. The study was a joint research venture by the American Association of Critical Care Nurses and VitalSmarts, an organizational leadership group, and explored the specific concerns people have regarding difficult communication that can contribute to avoidable errors and other chronic problems in healthcare. Fear of retaliation, concern about a breakdown in future work relationships, lack of time or opportunity to address the issue, and a failure to perceive it as one's job or duty to confront the unsafe behavior were among the reasons given.

The following are examples from the study:

A group of eight anesthesiologists agree a peer is dangerously incompetent, but they do not confront him. Instead, they go to great efforts to schedule surgeries for the sickest babies at times he is not on duty. This problem has persisted for over five years. (Focus Group of Physicians)

A group of nurses describe a peer as careless and inattentive. Instead of confronting her, they double check her work - sometimes running in to patient rooms to retake a blood pressure or redo a safety check. They've "worked around" this nurse's weaknesses for over a year. The nurses resent her, but never talk to her about their concerns. Nor do any of the doctors who also avoid and compensate for her. (Focus Group of Nurses)

Source: www.silencekills.com

**Letter from an RN in Response to "Silence Kills"**[15]

I was a nurse for 32 years, and in that time I witnessed several cases in which silence killed. I, too, have been guilty of not speaking up.

Four years ago, I started voicing my opinions - and immediately became the most unpopular nurse in my facility. Soon after, I left the field of nursing. I had witnessed the death of a 37-year-old caused by malpractice, denied a drunk surgeon access to an operating room - while other physicians refused to intervene - where he was going to perform surgery on a seven-year-old with a ruptured appendix, and have seen a physician insert a chest tube without sedation after a patient with a collapsed lung responded affirmatively to the physician's question of whether he smoked.

I understand nurses want to keep the peace and keep their jobs, but our silence is killing patients. We must offer help to the offenders, but the patient also needs protection - as does the nurse, who should be able to go home each night proud of her work.

*Name withheld upon request*

**Risk Management Strategies for the Chain of Command**
- Know your hospital's chain of command policy.
- The chain of command policy must be functional 24/7.
- Review it frequently.
- If a policy does not exist, be proactive in initiating one to be formulated.
- Timely response by team members must be ensured when there is a request for consultation and advice.
- Do not be afraid to initiate the chain of command when needed - remember that you are there for the patient.
- Document the process with the times and names of those notified and their responses.

### Failure to Provide Timely and Appropriate Newborn Resuscitation

Fetal status prior to birth has direct implications for the baby's condition at birth and the ability to plan for neonatal resuscitation. This assessment is a component of basic perinatal nursing care.[16] Nurses have been cited for not having the appropriate personnel readily available when a newborn needed resuscitation. It has been alleged that by not having the team assembled, precious moments are lost in resuscitating the newborn. Careful monitoring of the maternal condition during labor also will enable perinatal nurses to identify changes in maternal-fetal status. This allows the nurse to anticipate the needs of the neonate and notify the necessary personnel to attend the delivery.[3]

**Examples of Not Being Prepared for Infant Resuscitation**
#1  When baby boy Tommy was born, he took a breath, cried, moved his extremities, and opened his eyes. Dr. M. suctioned some fluid from Tommy's mouth and nose, cut the umbilical cord and turned him over to the delivery room nurse, Nurse T. Within approximately two to three minutes after delivery, the baby's condition started to deteriorate and he had trouble breathing.

Nurse T. suctioned some slightly bloody fluid from Tommy's stomach and forced oxygen into his lungs using positive pressure equipment.

Tommy did not respond and stopped breathing altogether. Dr. M. suctioned more fluid from the baby's stomach and then inserted an endotracheal tube into his windpipe. Before administering oxygen through the tube, he attempted to suction fluid from the baby's lungs by inserting a suction tube within the ET tube. The suction tube given to him by Nurse T. was too large to insert through the endotracheal tube. As a result, Dr. M. had to remove the endotracheal tube to suction Tommy's lungs and reinsert it to administer oxygen.

Tommy's condition continued to worsen, Dr. M. asked for an Ambu bag which he intended to attach to the ET tube, creating a closed system to maximize the flow of oxygen to the baby's lungs. He attempted without success to remove the mask from the Ambu bag. Nurse T. was asked to do it and was not able to. The Ambu could not be connected to the endotracheal tube.

The mask was then placed over the baby's mouth. The baby was severely cyanotic and becoming worse. Dr. M. started to blow air from his mouth into the ET tube. At 12 minutes of life, Tommy was breathing on his own. Tommy now is profoundly delayed with cerebral palsy.

The settlement was for nine million dollars. The nurse was found negligent in not having the necessary supplies available and for not being able to remove the mask from the Ambu bag. The hospital was held liable for not providing proper resuscitation equipment. The obstetrician was not found liable.

#2 A woman had a cesarean birth after prolonged labor without cervical change. When the baby was born approximately 45 minutes later, he was limp, blue, and without spontaneous respirations. Since a depressed baby was unexpected, the neonatal team was not asked to attend the birth. Resuscitation was difficult and the Apgar score at 10 minutes was 4. The baby was transferred to the NICU, requiring ventilator support for several hours. During a debriefing after the incident, it was noted that the fetal monitor had been removed in anticipation of an imminent transfer from the labor room to the OR; however, a more emergent case took priority, which caused delay. Fetal monitoring was not reinitiated, nor was fetal status assessed in the OR.[1]

---

**Risk Management Strategies for Staff to be Prepared for Neonatal Resuscitation**

- Follow guidelines for assessing the condition of the fetus right up until the time of delivery.
- There should always be at least one staff member whose primary responsibility is to the infant and who is qualified to begin resuscitation.
- Develop a list of maternal and fetal complications that require the presence in the delivery room of someone specifically qualified in all aspects of newborn resuscitation, including intubation and medication administration. Make sure all staff are familiar with this list. **See Table 3-2**.
- Develop a procedure to ensure the readiness of equipment and personnel and to provide for periodic review and evaluation of the effectiveness of the system.
- Contingency plans should be available for multiple births and other unusual circumstances.
- The resuscitation steps should be documented in the medical record with attention to accurate times.

Adapted from: AAP and ACOG (2007) Guidelines for Perinatal Care. 6th Ed.

---

**Failure to Appropriately Initiate Shoulder Dystocia Corrective Measures**

*"A sudden call to a gentlewoman in labor. The child's head delivered for a long time - but even with hard pulling from the midwife, the remarkably large shoulder prevented delivery. I have been called by midwives to many cases of this kind, in which the child was frequently lost."*

*Smellie, 1730*

Shoulder dystocia is an unpredictable obstetric emergency which requires prompt intervention in order to decrease risk of maternal-fetal trauma and long-term sequelae. Shoulder dystocias occur in about one percent of all deliveries, with the percentage rising for babies over 4,000g (10 percent) and 4,500g (20 percent). Brachial plexus injuries, in general, occur in 10 percent of all shoulder dystocia deliveries with 10 percent of these remaining permanent.[17]

Allegations have included failure to: accurately predict shoulder dystocia, diagnose labor abnormalities, appropriately initiate shoulder dystocia corrective maneuvers, perform a cesarean birth as well as applying forceps or vacuum at

**Table 3-2  Risk Factors Associated with the Need for Neonatal Resuscitation**

Antepartum Factors

| | |
|---|---|
| Maternal diabetes | Post-term gestation |
| Pregnancy-induced hypertension | Multiple gestation |
| Preeclampsia | Premature rupture of membranes |
| Chronic hypertension | Size-dates discrepancy |
| Fetal anemia or isoimmunization | Drug therapy, such as |
| Maternal cardiac, renal, pulmonary, thyroid or neurologic disease | Magnesium Sulfate |
| Previous fetal or neonatal death | adrenergic-blocking drugs |
| Bleeding in second or third trimester | Maternal substance abuse |
| Maternal infection | Fetal malformation or anomalies |
| No prenatal care | Decreased fetal activity |
| Fetal hydrops | Polyhydramnios |
| Age <16 or > 35 years | Oligohydramnios |

Intrapartum Factors

| | |
|---|---|
| Emergency cesarean section | Persistent bradycardia |
| Forceps or vacuum-assisted delivery | Non-reassuring fetal heart rate patterns |
| Breech or other abnormal presentation | General anesthesia |
| Premature labor | Uterine hyperstimulation |
| Precipitous labor | Narcotics administered to mother within 4 hours of delivery |
| Chorioamnionitis | Meconium-stained amniotic fluid |
| Prolonged rupture of membranes (>18 hours before delivery) | Prolapsed cord |

Prolonged labor (>24 hours)

Prolonged second stage of labor (>2 hours)

Macrosomia

Abruptio placentae

Placenta previa

Significant intrapartum bleeding

Used with permission of the American Heart Association & American Academy of Pediatrics. Neonatal Resuscitation Textbook. 5th edition. 2006. Copyright held by AAP.

*AHA & AAP suggest that a copy of these risk factors be posted in labor and delivery areas.*

high station or continued application without evidence of fetal descent resulting in shoulder dystocia and application of fundal pressure during shoulder dystocia further impacting the shoulder.[18]

---

**Risk Management Strategies In the Event of a Shoulder Dystocia**

❖ Since shoulder dystocia is unpredictable, assessment of the laboring patient cannot be overemphasized.

❖ Conduct frequent interdisciplinary shoulder dystocia drills on your unit.

❖ Each room should be equipped with a step stool.

❖ Practice maneuvers such as McRobert's and the proper positioning for suprapubic pressure.

❖ Remember that the physician or midwife is in charge - listen to their directions.

❖ Remain calm and support the patient.

❖ Make sure that a neonatal resuscitation team is in attendance - do not wait to call them.

❖ Document accurately: avoid documenting minute by minute account of the emergency unless it is absolutely certain that the times are accurate, attempt to closely approximate time interval between delivery of the fetal head and body, include fetal assessment data during the maneuvers, review EFM strip and talk with other providers in attendance to ensure that most accurate details of clinical circumstances are recorded and record attendance of newborn resuscitation team.[19] **Figure 3-3** is a checklist and worksheet which can be used to facilitate accurate documentation.

❖ Nurses should document only what was seen. Internal maneuvers and strength of traction are not data that anyone can document with certainty, except by the person performing them.[3]

---

**Take Home Message**

The prediction of shoulder dystocia is not within the scope of practice of the registered professional nurse; however, an awareness of maternal-fetal risks and being prepared to assist the CNM or physician if shoulder dystocia should occur is expected.

Source: Simpson, K.(1999). Shoulder Dystocia: Nursing Interventions and Risk Management Strategies. MCN The American Journal of Maternal/ Child Nursing. 24 (6). 305-311.

## Figure 3-3 Shoulder Dystocia Checklist and Worksheet

Date: _____

Attending MD: _____   CNM: _____

Resident MD: _____   Neo/Pedi: _____

Nurses: _____

Family member(s) present other than mother: _____

| PROCEDURE(S) PERFORMED: If attempted more than once, list time to begin and end each attempt | TIME | Time Begun | Time Ended |
|---|---|---|---|
| **DELIVERY OF HEAD** | | | |
| **CODE CALLED** | | | |
| **Arrival of Nursing** | | | |
| **Arrival of MD's** | | | |
| **Arrival of Other** (specify) | | | |
| Neo/Pedi | | | |
| Anesthesia | | | |
| **Episiotomy (unless prior to delivery)** | | | |
| **McRobert's** | | | |
| **Suprapubic Pressure** | | | |
| **Post. Arm Extraction** | | | |
| **Knee-Chest** | | | |
| **Wood's Corkscrew** | | | |
| **Transfer to OR** | | | |

(Use other side for more extensive note if necessary)

Delivery of infant: Time: _____   Birthweight: _____

Apgar: _____ @1 min   _____ @ 5 min   _____ @ 10 min

**Immediate infant assessment:**   **No apparent injury** _____

Circle:

Suspect clavicle fx   **right**   **left**   Suspect humerus fx   **right**   **left**

Movement of right arm:   absent   minimal   active

Movement of left arm:   absent   minimal   active

Baby transferred to:   normal newborn nursery   NICU   Other: _____

Additional items:  Please check if done.

_____ Immediate discussion with family documented

_____ **Delivery team reviewed time frames and procedures prior to entering them into the medical record**

_____ Detailed delivery note or dictation - signed/dated/timed

_____ Incident Report filed &/or Risk Management notified if applicable

**\*\*\*\*\*Remember that this is a Worksheet/Checklist and does not become part of the permanent record.**

## Common Alleged Deviations from the Standard of Nursing Care & Risk Management

**The Concept of Failure to Rescue**

Failure to rescue is an indicator that has been used to measure quality of care in the in-patient setting for surgical patients by evaluating the number of patients who die after developing postoperative complications which were not present on admission. It is based on the premise that although deaths in hospitals are sometimes unavoidable, many can be prevented.[13, 20] It must also be acknowledged that opportunities to identify complications and to intervene when they occur are sometimes lost. The more deaths there are at a hospital among patients with complications, the more likely there were problems with the process of care in that hospital. Research has shown that the failure-to-rescue rate is a better indicator of a hospital's quality of care than is the rate of complications alone.[20]

Geller[21] and colleagues have reported that the probability of a woman progressing along the morbidity/mortality continuum was significantly related to whether she had a preventable event. The results showed that this association was specifically due to provider factors, incomplete or inappropriate management, as opposed to system or patient factors. They felt that this was critically important because it means that changes in provider decision-making could reduce the severity of disease experienced by high-risk women.

There are 2 key components of failure to rescue: (a) careful surveillance and timely identification of complications and (b) taking action by quickly initiating appropriate interventions and activating a team response. The perinatal population, though not previously considered, presents direct implications for perinatal safety and lessons to be learned.[13] Using a non-reassurng fetal heart pattern and the importance of initiating intrauterine resuscitative measures as an example, Simpson recommends[22] avoiding using outcomes as the only measurement end-point; rather, evaluate processes including timeliness and the quality of the perinatal team's response to a nonreassuring heart rate tracing. A systematic evaluation of the perinatal team's response using the key components of the concept of failure to rescue, with subsequent changes in practice and teamwork dynamics based on the findings, can potentially avoid a preventable adverse outcome when complications and/or emergent situations arise in the future.

Maternal and fetal complications and emergencies which are appropriate for evaluation based on the concept of failure to rescue include:[13]

**Maternal**
➢ Placental abruption
➢ Uterine rupture

74

> ➢ Magnesium sulfate toxicity
> ➢ Eclampsia
> ➢ Post partum hemorrhage

**Fetal**

> ➢ Nonreassuring fetal heart rate pattern
> ➢ Prolapsed umbilical cord
> ➢ Uterine hyperstimulation
> ➢ Second stage fetal intolerance to pushing
> ➢ Shoulder dystocia
> ➢ Emergent cesarean birth for nonreassuring fetal status

Since nurses spend the majority of time with the patient, it is the nurse who is most likely the first to recognize signs of possible complications. The nurse's role in alerting the team and mobilizing its response has a direct impact on the ultimate outcome. Adequate staffing, staff mix and the ability to mobilize hospital resources quickly are crucial to rescuing the patient and preventing worsening of their condition. However, no matter the number of competent nurses, the clinical environment must support the nurse to bring the primary provider to the bedside when necessary and to set in motion a series of interventions to provide timely treatment.[20] The status of the nurses in the hospital, as evidenced by the respect of their physician colleagues and support from administrators, influences their ability to effect a successful rescue.[20]

---

**Example of Failure to Rescue**

Mrs. Jones, G 1 P0, was admitted at 3 a.m. with a history of having ruptured her membranes and experiencing irregular contractions. She is 40 2/7 weeks gestation. Her prenatal history is significant for gestational diabetes which has been controlled with insulin. Her exam on admission was 1 cm/70%/-1. It is now 11 a.m. and a vaginal exam is done which reveals the cervix to be 6 cm/100%. The presenting part is still at -1 station. She has epidural anesthesia and is comfortable. The fetal monitor shows a FHBL of 140 with moderate variability and occasional variable decelerations which respond to position change. Contractions are every 3-4 minutes, lasting 50 seconds and are moderate when palpated. The physician orders Pitocin to be started according to protocol. You start the Pitocin, effective contractions are established and the patient becomes fully dilated at 4 p.m. The presenting part is now at 0 station and she starts to push. After one hour of pushing, the station is still 0 station and variable decelerations are seen with every contraction. You carry out intrauterine resuscitative measures with little improvement. Variability is moderate. The patient is becoming

---

tired and having difficulty effectively pushing. You notify the M.D. who examines the patient. The cervix is slightly edematous on the right side and the station is now +1. You have the patient push while on her left side. After another hour, the M.D. reports that the vertex is at +1-+2. The FHR is now 160 with minimal variability. The Pitocin continues and the patient attempts to push with each contraction. At 8 p.m. (after 4 hours of pushing) the M.D. attempts a vacuum extraction since the FHR is now 180 with minimal variability and late and variable decelerations are present. The vacuum is applied 6 times with 4 pop-offs noted. You are having difficulty tracing the FHR. There is no descent noted and a STAT cesarean section is called. A baby boy weighing 4500 grams is delivered with Apgars of 3 at one minute, 6 at 5 minutes and 7 at 10 minutes.

1. Mahlmeister L. The perinatal nurse's role in obstetric emergencies: Legal issues and practice issues in the era of health care redesign. *J Perinat Neonat Nurs.* 1996; 10:32-46.

2. Helm A. *Nursing Malpractice: Sidestepping Legal Minefields.* Philadelphia: Lippincott,Williams & Wilkins; 2003.

3. Dunn PA, Gies ML, Peters MA. Perinatal litigation and related nursing issues. *Clinics in Perinatology.* 2005; 32:277-290.

4. Rostant D, Cady R. *Liability Issues in Perinatal Nursing.* Philadelphia: Lippincott; 1999.

5. Federico F. Responding to a medication error. *Forum.* 2003; 23:18.

6. Simpson KR, Knox EG. Risk management and electronic fetal monitoring: Decreasing risk of adverse outcomes and liability exposure. *J Perinat Neonat Nurs.* 2000; 14:40-52.

7. Cherouny PH, Federico FA, Haraden C, Leavitt Gullo S, Resar R. Idealized design of perinatal care. IHI innovation series white paper. Cambridge, Massachusetts: Institution for Healthcare Improvement; 2005. Available from: www.IHI.org.

8. Ives-Erikson J, Clifford J. Building a foundation for nurse-physician collaboration. *Forum.* 2008; 2:6-7.

9. Benner P, Sheets V, Uris P, Malloch K, Schwed K, Jamison D. Individual, practice, and system causes of errors in nursing: A taxonomy. *J Nurs Adm.* 2002; 32:509-523.

10. Goldberg K, ed. *Surefire Documentation: How,What, and When Nurses Need to Document.* St.Louis: Mosby; 1999.

11. Greenwald LM, Mondor M. Malpractice and the perinatal nurse. *J Perinat Neonat Nurs.* 2003; 17:101-109.

12. Joint Commission on Accreditation of Health Care Organizations. Effectively using chain-of-command policies. *Joint Commission Perspectives in Patient Safety.* 2005; 5:5-6.

13. Simpson KR. Failure to rescue: Implications for evaluating quality of care during labor and birth. *J Perinat Neonat Nurs.* 2005; 19:24-36.

14. Simpson K, Creehan P. *Perinatal Nursing.* 3rd ed. Philadelphia: Lippincott Williams & Wilkins:; 2008.

15. Allen DE. The code of silence. *Am J Nurs.* 2004; 104:85-86.

16. Simpson KR. Assessing fetal well-being prior to cesarean birth. *MCN: The American Journal of Maternal/Child Nursing.* 2007; 32:328-330.

17. Lerner H. Three typical claims in shoulder dystocia lawsuits. *Forum.* 2007; 25:15-17.

18. Simpson KR, Knox GE. Common areas of litigation related to care during labor and birth: Recommendations to promote patient safety and decrease risk exposure. *J Perinat Neonat Nurs.* 2003; 17:110-127.
19. Simpson KR. Shoulder dystocia: Nursing interventions and risk-management strategies. *MCN* 1999; 24:305-311.
20. Clarke SP, Aiken LH. Failure to rescue: Needless deaths are prime examples of the need for more nurses at the bedside. *Am J Nurs.* 2003; 103:42-47.
21. Geller SE, Rosenberg D, Cox SM, et al. The continuum of maternal morbidity and mortality: Factors associated with severity. *Am J Obstet Gynecol.* 2004; 191:939-944.
22. Simpson KR. Failure to rescue in obstetrics. *MCN Am J Matern Child Nurs.* 2005; 30:76.

# CHAPTER 4

# The Power of Documentation

At a recent conference sponsored by Harvard Risk Management, a defense attorney shared his experience of how the topic he had chosen to present had come about. In preparation for his talk, he had gone to a colleague and asked him what he thought the audience would most benefit from. The suggestion was made that he address documentation. Not satisfied with this answer (he thought it would be too boring), he queried three more colleagues and received the same answer each time - DOCUMENTATION, DOCUMENTATION, DOCUMENTATION. There is no getting around it; the importance of documentation of patient care cannot be over emphasized.

Patients are often cared for by large multidisciplinary teams (doctors, nurses, therapists, social workers, pharmacists) and accurate documentation may be the patient's only protection against fragmented care. The written record links clinicians to one another. Poor documentation of care not only impedes communication among providers, but often complicates defense against malpractice claims. Incomplete or absent documentation may be interpreted as indicating a lack of planning for a particular course of action, and gaps in documentation make it difficult to determine the rationale behind a decision. Another potential problem with documentation can occur when the medical record contains contradictory statements, due to differences in interpretation, recorded by different providers.

When the miscommunication is between a physician and a nurse, it can give rise to conflicts of interest significant enough to alter the defense of the case. When the evidence to be presented at trial will make the presentation of a unified defense difficult (if not impossible), cases that would otherwise be defensible have to be settled, usually with both the physician and the nurse contributing to the settlement amount.[2] Remember that from a legal perspective, there is an argument that, if it wasn't documented, it wasn't done; if it was poorly documented, it was poorly done; and if it was incorrectly documented, it was fraudulent. Quality writing inspires confidence in quality performance.[3 P-105]

Documentation of nursing care must meet the standard of the profession. Documentation that meets these standards provides a factual and objective account of both direct and indirect communication of the patient's status, medical treatment and nursing care. By being conscientious of the standard of care, providing the nursing care based on the standard of care and documenting that care you are protecting both your patient and yourself. Also, nurses are ethically and legally accountable to all of their patients. The scope of your professional responsibility is set out by your state's Nurse Practice Act and by other state and federal regulations. Documenting the nursing care provided in the patient's medical record is one way of accepting that responsibility and of being accountable to the patient and your profession.[4]

Standards of care set minimum criteria for your proficiency on the job, enabling others to judge the quality of care you and your nursing colleagues provide. Some nurses regard standards of nursing care as impractical ideals that have little or no bearing on the reality of working life. This is a dangerous misconception. You are expected to meet the standards of nursing care for every nursing task that you perform.[3] Documentation of the nursing care you provide is essential to the credibility that your care meets the standard of care a patient might expect from a prudent nurse in a similar situation. Even when late entries must be made (and in case of emergencies this is the most likely method of charting), the nurse must detail all affirmative duty actions.[5] During a deposition or trial a nurse might have the opportunity to present additional information, although a jury may not consider undocumented evidence as strongly as contemporaneous documentation in the medical record.[6]

**Principles of Good Documentation**

The American Nurses Association (ANA), the Joint Commission on Accreditation of Healthcare Organizations (JCAHO) and the Centers for Medicare and Medicaid Services have established that documentation must include ongoing assessment, variations from the assessment, patient teaching, responses to therapy, and relevant statements made by the patient.[4] In obstetrics, certain known complications are not predictable; therefore, clinicians must be more diligent about documenting thorough assessments and events contemporaneously when possible.[7]

Nursing documentation is varied, complex, and time consuming. Studies reflect that nurses spend from 35 to 140 minutes on charting per shift. Logically, the severity of the patient's condition should determine charting time: in reality, however, the nurse spends the most time in repetitive, duplicative charting of routine care and observations. As a result, too often specific significant observations or dialogues are not recorded because of time constraints. Moreover, significant information that is recorded may be missed because nurses and doctors do not regularly read nurses' progress notes.[8]

Documentation (regardless of the system used) should reflect:
➤ Time and date
➤ The nursing process - assessment, nursing diagnosis, outcome identification, planning, implementation, and evaluation
➤ Factual, accurate and complete information

➤ Objectivity - chart only what you see, hear, smell and do.

➤ Timely communication - evidence must be present that communication with the physician or midwife has been made when any change in the patient's condition warrants it. *Physician notified* is not enough. Write what you reported to the physician and the response.

➤ Appropriate documentation of late entries. Date and time when you are writing the note as well as the date and time the event occurred. **Remember a late entry is better than no entry**.[9]

➤ Avoidance of block charting as it covers too much time and a patient's attorney may contend that you failed to render timely care or that too much time elapsed between your detection of a problem and its correction. Always record the date and time of each entry and the date and exact times for specific assessment findings, interventions, and other actions.[9]

➤ Legible notes

➤ Consistency

➤ Corrections are made appropriately - a single line is drawn through the words to be corrected, signed and dated.

➤ Approved hospital abbreviations

➤ The signature of the person rendering the care including first and last name and professional licensure

➤ *Always* do your own charting. Never let someone else document the care you give or do not chart for someone else.

➤ Read documentation carefully before you countersign another person's notes

➤ Understand and follow the documentation standards of your facility and state[3]

➤ All teaching including the patient's understanding of what has been taught

➤ Chart procedures when you do them - never in advance

**Affirmative Duty Documentation**

When the nurse is confronted with an obstetric complication or emergency that requires a health care team management approach, the nursing notes must reflect prompt, appropriate, affirmative duty actions:[5]

➤ Who the nurse notified:
  • Name and title of the person notified.
➤ What the nurse reported:
  • Significant data.
  • Changes in the patient status.

> ➤ What the nurse requested:
>   - Examination or assessment of the patient or data already obtained.
>   - Specific health care provider (MD, CNM, RN).
>   - Equipment, supplies, or medications.
>   - Other types of help (telephone calls, assistance with moving the patient).
> ➤ What the response to or outcome of the nurse's request was:
>   - The time when people arrived.
>   - The time when examinations or assessments were performed.
>   - Any new orders given.
>   - Any new plan made with health team members.

Due to the scope of this book, all available methods of documentation cannot be addressed. However, five of the most common types of documentation systems, with their pluses and minuses, are included in **TABLE 4-1**. Nurses should avoid using forms with preprinted times and limited space for notations. These types of forms lead to inherently inaccurate or inadequate documentation. Vital signs and other maternal-fetal assessments or emergencies do not occur at predetermined 15-minute intervals. There are times when more comprehensive documentation is required than can fit into limited, preset boxes.[10]

The most important thing to remember, no matter what method of documentation you use, is that nursing documentation is the only evidence that nursing assessments were carried out, physician orders were implemented, the nursing process was utilized, patient's responses were evaluated, communication took place with the physician and other health care providers, and standards were maintained.[11 P-30]

**Table 4-1  Types of Documentation Systems**

| Documentation System | Pluses | Minuses |
|---|---|---|
| **Problem oriented:**<br>Based on assessment findings, team members create a problem list, formulate an initial plan of care for each problem, use multidisciplinary notes, and write a discharge summary that tells whether each problem was resolved. The acronym SOAP is typically used;<br>**S**ubjective data - what the patient says<br>**O**bjective - information gathered through physical examination<br>**A**ssessment - analysis based on subjective and objective data<br>**P**lan - actions to be implemented | Organizes information into specific categories<br>Illustrates the continuity of care<br>Promotes documentation of the nursing process<br>Facilitates more consistent documentation<br>Eliminates documentation of non essential data<br>Potentially serves as a checklist that draws attention to problems requiring intervention | Need to know the format<br>Can be repetitious of assessment findings and interventions<br>Emphasizes problems so that routine care may remain undocumented unless flowsheets are also used<br>Difficulties may arise if staff fail to update the problem list regularly<br>Not well suited for settings with rapid patient turnover |
| **Narrative Notes**<br>Traditional narrative charting systems document ongoing assessment data, nursing interventions, and patient responses in chronological order | Easy to learn.<br>Can be used in any clinical setting<br>Combine nicely with flowsheets so as to decrease charting time | Can be repetitive and time consuming<br>Reflect the author's subjective viewpoint<br>Do not allow easy tracking of problems and trends<br>May seem disorganized |

| | Advantages | Disadvantages |
|---|---|---|
| **Charting by Exception**<br>Requires documentation only of significant or abnormal findings.<br>Established guidelines for assessments and interventions must be adhered to | Decreases documentation time<br>Eliminates redundancies<br>Clearly identifies abnormal data<br>The use of well-defined guidelines and standards of care promotes uniform nursing practice | Do not always reflect the nursing process<br>Potentially vague<br>Major time commitment needed to develop clear guidelines and standards of care<br>To ensure a legally sound patient record, these guidelines *must* be in place and understood by all nursing staff *before* the format can be implemented<br>Does not accommodate integrated or multidisciplinary charting<br>Unexpected events or isolated occurrences may not be fully documented<br>System was developed for RNs/ if LPNs use the system, it must be evaluated and modified so that it meets their scope of practices |
| **Computerized Charting** | Reduces documentation time<br>Complete nurse management reports may be obtained<br>Provides patient classification data<br>Identifies patient-teaching needs<br>Supplies data for nursing research and | Computer downtimes<br>There are many nurses who are not familiar with using a computer<br>Inaccurate or incomplete information can occur if standardized, limited vocabulary or phrases are used. |

| | | |
|---|---|---|
| | education<br>Multidisciplinary access<br>Legibility<br>Remote access<br>Access to clinical information<br>Patient driven care planning<br>Nursing information systems can increase efficiency and accuracy in all phases of the nursing process | |
| **Flow Sheets** | Displays a specific aspect of care (i.e. Vital signs)<br>Saves time/ quick and easy<br>Documents continuous care | Space is limited<br>Duplication of information when combined with a narrative note<br>May be treated too casually<br>May not reflect complete care if not accompanied by a narrative note – a narrative note should be written when you need to clarify something and show that you took appropriate action<br>A policy must be in place describing how blank spaces are to be addressed (a blank space may imply that a full assessment was not done) |

> **Example of a "No-Win" Situation When a Nurse Does Not Document the Substance of a Conversation Requesting a Physician Come to the Bedside[11 P-115]**
>
> Consider this scenario. A physician refuses the request of a nurse to come to the hospital to assess a patient and fetal monitor tracing. The nurse does not document the substance of the conversation or even if the call took place. If there is a lawsuit, the nurse will be questioned as to whether she interpreted the fetal heart tracing as abnormal and the following will transpire:
> - ➤ If she did interpret the tracing as abnormal, then clearly she deviated from the standard of care by failing to communicate the information to the physician.
> - ➤ If she did communicate the information and the physician refused to attend to the patient, the nurse would be negligent in not implementing the chain of command.
> - ➤ If the nurse did not interpret the strip as abnormal, then she is negligent in her interpretation of the strip.

## The Nursing Process & Critical Thinking

Nurses have long been taught to use the nursing process to guide their practice.[12 P-116] The five steps of the nursing process are assessment, diagnosis, planning, implementation, and evaluation. This process provides a framework for identifying and treating the patient's problems. The nursing process is an ongoing and interactive cycle that results in flexible, individualized, and dynamic nursing care for all patients. Assessment is the foundation of the process and leads to the identification of both nursing diagnoses and collaborative problems. Nursing diagnosis provides the primary focus for developing patient specific individualization of patient goals. The planning process allows for individualization of patient goals and nursing care within the context of managed care guidelines. Implementation involves providing nursing actions to treat each diagnosis. Ongoing evaluation determines the degree of success in achieving the client's goals and the continued relevance of each nursing diagnosis and collaborative problem.[12 P-121]

Following the nursing process requires critical thinking. The need for critical thinking in nursing has greatly increased with the diversity and complexity of nursing practice. A nurse working in a special care unit is typically subject to the general rule of law as her staff nurse colleagues: She must meet the standard of care that a reasonably prudent nurse would meet in the same or similar circumstances. However, in a malpractice lawsuit, when deciding whether a specialty nurse has acted reasonably, the court will not consider what the average registered nurse or licensed practical nurse would have done, but rather what they were specifically trained to do.[3 P-98]

Perinatal nurses must be critical thinkers because of the nature of the discipline and their work. Perinatal nurses are frequently confronted with problem situations: critical thinking enables them to make sound decisions. These decisions often determine the well-being of patients and even their survival. The decisions must be sound. Critical thinking skills are needed to assess information and plan decisions. When unexpected complications arise, critical thinking ability helps nurses to recognize important cues, respond quickly, and adapt interventions to specific needs.

**TABLE 4-2** illustrates how the nursing process is used in perinatal nursing for a patient who presents to the triage area complaining of abdominal cramping at 32 weeks gestation.

**Table 4-2**

| Nursing Process | Critical Thinking Skills | Example |
|---|---|---|
| ***Assessment*** Involves specific activities of gathering, substantiating, and communicating data that, together, provide a comprehensive view of a person's health status. | Observing Distinguishing relevant from irrelevant Distinguishing important from unimportant data Validating data Organizing data Categorizing data | The nurse would: Access and review the patient's prenatal record Identify gravida, para, EDC Question the patient as to: <ul><li>time the cramping started</li><li>description of the cramping including location and level of pain using a scale of 0-10</li><li>association with bleeding or leaking of fluid, nausea, vomiting or diarrhea</li><li>possible injury (MVA, fall, domestic violence)</li></ul> Vital signs Vaginal exam per RN or provider depending on situation Establish fetal well-being/presence or absence of contractions |
| ***Analysis/diagnosis*** A nursing diagnosis is a statement that the nurse makes about an actual or potential nursing care need of a patient. | Finding patterns and relationships Making inferences Stating the problem Suspending judgment | Risk for pre term delivery |

| | | |
|---|---|---|
| **Planning**<br>Identification of nursing actions or nursing interventions required to prevent, reduce, or eliminate the nursing diagnoses identified during the diagnostic phase. | Generalizing Transferring knowledge from one situation to another<br>Developing evaluative criteria<br>Hypothesizing | Continue to evaluate vital signs<br>Continue to monitor fetal well-being/ contractions via electronic fetal monitoring<br>Continue to assess pain level<br>Communicate findings to the healthcare provider, obtain orders and carry out<br>Should delivery seem imminent notify other personnel (anesthesia, NICU) and activate resources (other RNs)<br>Support the patient and keep her and her companion apprised of the situation |
| **Implementation**<br>Actual delivery of the nursing care phase of the nursing process. | Applying knowledge<br>Testing hypotheses | Carry out plan as outlined |
| **Evaluation**<br>Review of goal achievement and reassessment of nursing actions. | Deciding whether hypotheses are correct<br>Making criterion-based evaluations and judgments | If imminent delivery, all personnel are assembled and patient is safely delivered of pre term infant. Appropriate care is rendered to infant without delay. |

Adapted from: Nunnery, R (1997). Advancing your career: Concepts of professional nursing. F. A. Davis: Philadelphia

**Preventing ASSESSMENT Documentation ERRORS**

*The most important practical lesson that can be given to nurses is to teach them what to observe - how to observe - what symptoms indicate improvement - what the reverse - which are of importance - which are of none - which are evidence of neglect - and of what kind of neglect. All of this is what ought to make part, and an, essential part, of the training of every nurse.*

*Florence Nightingale, Notes on Nursing 1859*

Except on special units or unless a physician orders otherwise, nurses routinely assess patients every two to four hours; in the case of an unstable patient, a diligent nurse assesses the patient even more frequently. Any gap in nursing documentation of several hours or more can be a red flag to a jury. The standards of nursing care include documenting the patient's condition at the time of each assessment, even if it is unchanged or stable.[13]

When documenting, be sure to address the following:

- What is a normal assessment for this patient at this time?
- Is the patient's current assessment different from the previous assessments?
- If the assessment is different, how is it different? Is it better or worse?
- What will the next nurse need to know to better understand and care for the patient?

**Table 4-3** outlines the guidelines for maternal - fetal assessments during labor and delivery and maternal-newborn assessments during the immediate postpartum period.

**Preventing INTERVENTION Documentation ERRORS**

Intervention errors in nursing documentation might consist of failure to follow up with the physician in a timely manner, fulfill physician orders, or move up the chain of command if the physician's orders or actions are endangering the patient.[11] In my experience of reviewing medical records in which documentation is an issue, I have found the lack of documentation of intrauterine resuscitative measures to be most egregious. In deposition, the nurse will often state that doing intrauterine resuscitative measures is her norm; however, they are not documented. This makes it virtually impossible for the nursing expert to support the nursing care when documentation does not exist. Often when intrauterine resuscitative measures have been documented, it has also been my experience, that the omission of documentation of the nurse having notified the provider and/or the conversation that ensued is most prevalent.

**Table 4-3  Guidelines for Maternal-Fetal Assessments During Labor and Birth and Maternal-Newborn Assessments During the Immediate Postpartum Period**

| Hospital Admission of Pregnant Women | Immediate Postpartum Period | Newborn Assessments |
|---|---|---|
| The following (at minimum) need to be assessed whenever a pregnant woman presents to a hospital regardless of whether the complaint is pregnancy-related or not: <br><br> • Fetal heart rate <br> • Maternal vital signs <br> • Uterine contractions <br><br> The responsible obstetric care provider should be promptly informed if any of the following are present: <br><br> • Vaginal bleeding <br> • Acute abdominal pain <br> • Temperature of >100.4 <br> • Preterm labor <br> • Preterm premature rupture of membranes <br> • Hypertension <br><br> The following are to be assessed and documented during the admission for labor: <br> Date and time of the woman's arrival <br> Date and time of the provider's notification <br><br> • Pain level <br> • Vital signs <br> • Fetal heart rate <br> • Contraction pattern including frequency, duration and intensity | Immediately post delivery: <br><br> • Vital signs (B/P & Pulse) every 15 minutes for the first hour/ <br> • Temperature every 4 hours <br> • Fundus - firmness & position <br> • Lochia - amount, color, odor <br> • Level of pain and response to medication <br> • Response to delivery <br> • Bonding with newborn <br><br> Hospital policies should be written addressing frequency and criteria for assessments during the mother's hospital stay. | Apgar scores should be obtained at 1 and 5 minutes and for an extended period of time until the Apgar score is 7 or >. <br> During the stabilization period the following is assessed and documented every 30 minutes until the newborn has been stable for 30 minutes: <br><br> • Temperature <br> • Pulse <br> • Respiratory rate and type <br> • Tone <br> • Color <br> • Activity <br><br> Continued observation for any of the following signs of illness should be done and reported to the provider: <br><br> • Temperature instability <br> • Change in activity, refusal of feedings <br> • Unusual skin color <br> • Abnormal cardiac or respiratory rate and rhythm <br> • Delayed or abnormal stools or voiding <br> • Abdominal distention, bilious vomiting <br> • Excessive lethargy and sleeping |

- Time the contractions started
- Presence of fetal movement
- Membrane status
- Vaginal exam results
- Estimated fetal weight
- Fetal presentation and station
- Urine protein and glucose
- Risk factors
- History of allergies
- Time of last ingested food and drink
- Medications including over the counter medications and herbs
- Time medications were last used
- History of drug, alcohol and cigarette use
- History of domestic violence
- Birthing Plan

Labor and Birth

- Maternal vitals per hospital protocol and at least every 4 hours. This may be increased according to the patient's status.
- Fetal Heart Rate

  No risk factors:

  ➢ At least every 30 minutes during the active phase of the first stage of labor/ and at least every 15 minutes during the second stage of labor

  Risk factors present:

  ➢ During the active phase if auscultation is used, the FHR should be evaluated and recorded every 15 minutes after a uterine contraction/with EFM – the

➤ tracing should be evaluated every 15 minutes

➤ During the second stage, the FHR should be evaluated every 5 minutes

Uterine Activity
- Evaluation per hospital protocol

Labor Progress
- Vaginal examinations should assess dilation, effacement and station of the presenting part

Additional Parameters
- Characteristics of amniotic fluid: amount, color, odor
- Characteristics bloody show/bleeding
- Maternal response to labor
- Effectiveness of pain management
- Effectiveness of partner support

Adapted from: American Academy of Pediatrics and American College of Obstetricians and Gynecologists (2002). Guidelines for perinatal care (5th ed.), Elk Grove Village, IL: Author; Association of Women's Health, Obstetric and Neonatal Nurses. (1998). Standards and guidelines for professional nursing practice in care of women and newborns (5th ed.) Washington, DC: author.

**Failure to Intervene**
**Fairfax Hospital System, Inc. v McCarty (1992)**

Mrs. McCarty was 31 years old when she was admitted to Fairfax Hospital to deliver her first child. Mrs. McCarty was placed on an electronic fetal monitor at about 7:30 A.M. after spontaneous rupture of membranes. A nurse began attending to her about 6:10 P.M. that evening and was to be with her until 9:00 P.M. The evidence presented in court established that the fetal heart rate monitor demonstrated a broad-based deceleration at approximately 8:27 P.M. The mother began demonstrating an abnormal labor pattern and the fetal heart rate monitor demonstrated that the fetus was experiencing more and more difficulty. In spite of the fetal distress apparent on the fetal monitor strip as early as 8:27 P.M., the nurse did not notify the physician until 8:50 P.M. The obstetrician, testifying for the plaintiffs, indicated that the nurse did not tell him an emergency situation was present. He testified that a cesarean delivery could have been accomplished within 12 minutes and that had he seen the fetal monitor, he would have moved to deliver the infant shortly before 8:40 P.M. The obstetrician further testified that the nurse's failure to take action or notify him delayed delivery and contributed to the eventual outcome of the infant. The infant has severe neurological impairments.
Settlement: $3.5 million dollars.

**Take Home Message**

Failure to follow the rules of good documentation can and has made the difference in jury decisions. Keep in mind that the chart can be your friend or foe and is the best evidence of what you did or might not have done for your patient. When in doubt, DOCUMENT!

1. Cherouny PH, Federico FA, Haraden C, Leavitt Gullo S, Resar R. Idealized design of perinatal care. IHI innovation series white paper. Cambridge, Massachusetts: Institution for Healthcare Improvement; 2005. Available from: www.IHI.org.
2. Hunter C. Lessons from settled malpractice cases involving failed physician-nurse communication. *Forum.* 2008; 2:8-9.
3. Helm A. *Nursing Malpractice: Sidestepping Legal Minefields.* Philadelphia: Lippincott, Williams & Wilkins; 2003.
4. Holmes H, ed. *Complete Guide to Documentation.* Philadelphia: Lippincott; 2003.
5. Mahlmeister L. The perinatal nurse's role in obstetric emergencies: Legal issues and practice issues in the era of health care redesign. *J Perinat Neonat Nurs.* 1996; 10:32-46.
6. Dunn PA, Gies ML, Peters MA. Perinatal litigation and related nursing issues. *Clinics in Perinatology.* 2005; 32:277-290.
7. Rubeor K. The role of risk management in maternal-child health. *J Perinat Neonat Nurs.* 2003; 17:94-100.
8. Carpenito L. Documentation of nursing care. In: *Nursing Care Plans & Documentation.* 2nd ed. Philadelphia: Lippincott; 1999.
9. Goldberg K, ed. *Surefire Documentation: How, What, and When Nurses Need to Document.* St.Louis: Mosby; 1999.
10. Simpson K, Creehan P. *Perinatal Nursing.* 3rd ed. Philadelphia: Lippincott Williams & Wilkins: 2008.
11. Rostant D, Cady R. *Liability Issues in Perinatal Nursing.* Philadelphia: Lippincott; 1999.
12. Nunnery R. *Advancing Your Career: Concepts of Professional Nursing.* Philadelphia: F.A. Davis; 1997.
13. Ferrell KG. Documentation, part 2: The best evidence of care. Complete and accurate charting can be crucial to exonerating nurses in civil lawsuits. *Am J Nurs.* 2007; 107:61-64.

# CHAPTER 5

# Electronic Fetal Monitoring

*There is a need to develop clear guidelines for fetal monitoring of potential high-risk patients including nursing protocols for the interpretation of fetal rate tracings and to educate nurses, residents, nurse midwives and physicians to use standard terminology to communicate abnormal fetal heart tracings.*

*Sentinel Event Alert, Issue #30,*
*Preventing Infant Death and Injury During Delivery*

**Overview of Electronic Fetal Monitoring**

Electronic Fetal Monitoring (EFM) was introduced in the 1960s and is used to assess fetal status during labor. Despite the 2005 recommendation[1] of the American College of Obstetrics and Gynecology to limit the use of continuous fetal heart rate monitoring, the electronic fetal monitor is central to most labor and delivery units today. The use of electronic fetal heart rate monitoring is generally quoted as 80% in North America, but it is probable that almost all pregnant mothers have at least some EFM either before or during labor.[2]

The original rationale for the introduction of EFM was that it could serve as a screening test for asphyxia that is severe enough to cause neurologic damage or fetal death. That is, it could allow the recognition of asphyxia at a sufficiently early stage so that timely obstetric intervention would avoid asphyxiation-induced brain damage or death. When EFM was developed and introduced into clinical practice, it was hoped that it would lead to a reduction in the overall incidence of cerebral palsy which was believed to be due to birth asphyxia. It is now known that the majority of cases of infant and childhood cerebral palsy are related to events remote from labor and birth. In 10 developing countries, including the United States, despite a fivefold increase in cesarean deliveries over recent decades, driven in part by fetal monitoring, the incidence of cerebral palsy has remained steady at about 1 in 500 births, with similar rates around the world.[3] In part, the difficulty in distinguishing benign variant patterns from patterns associated with significant fetal acidemia arose because FHR monitoring was introduced into clinical practice before the cause of FHR patterns was well understood. Two aspects of FHR physiology, FHR variability and pattern evolution over time, were not addressed to any significant degree.[4-6]

Continuous or intermittent fetal heart monitoring tracings provide a convenient and reasonably predictable way of assessing fetal well-being. It also provides a current and continuous observation of indirect, subjective information about fetal oxygenation at the time the monitoring is being done. It does not explain oxygenation in the past or predict the future oxygenation during fetal life in the same way we once expected.[7] Fetal heart rate interpretation, although based on sound, scientific principles, is nonetheless an art with a subjective component. Although there is usually consensus regarding the more common fetal heart rate patterns, it is not unusual for interpreters to disagree. Different educational backgrounds, experiences, and clinical skills can result in wide variations in interpretations between experienced nurses and physicians. Communication issues and professional disagreements regarding EFM interpretation are much more likely to occur when attempting to assign a diagnosis of fetal compromise than that of fetal well-being.[6, 8]

## National Institute of Child and Human Development (NICHD) Nomenclature

In 1997, an interdisciplinary team of expert physicians and nurses was brought together by the National Institute of Health to address the major impediment to progress in the evaluation and investigation of FHR monitoring due to a lack of agreement in definitions and nomenclature.

Prior to that, there was no single standard, unambiguous set of definitions; physician and nursing literature typically referenced differing nomenclature for describing FHR patterns seen on electronic fetal monitors. Most nurses and doctors acquired their EFM skills through on-the–job training rather than as a formal didactic education.[9] As a result of that meeting, the National Institute of Child Health and Human Development Research Planning Workshop standardized principles for the basis of defining terms and their interpretive value in assessing fetal heart rate tracings.[5] This is known as NICHD nomenclature and is being incorporated into professional education programs for physicians, midwives and nurses. The benefits of a standardized nomenclature include:[10]

> ➢ Communication: clinicians now have a single, objective, and definitive set of terms to use when communicating with each other regarding FHR monitoring. Documentation can also be standardized
> ➢ Promotion of meaningful interpretation of FHR research, by standardizing the terms researchers use as well as clinicians use to describe FHR patterns and variability
> ➢ Legally - clinicians and experts repeatedly fail to give the same information when questioned by attorneys. (Standardization of terminology will help us all to be on the same page.)

Highly reliable perinatal teams have adopted the NICHD language and train nurses and obstetricians together. During the training, differences in interpretation are addressed and consensus is obtained regarding the desired action or response to specific interpretations.[11]

**Guidelines for Assessment and Management of Fetal Heart Rate Patterns**

Despite numerous attempts in the past 30 years, the obstetric community has been unable to reach a broad consensus on a standardized approach to the management of most fetal heart rate monitoring patterns. There are no universally accepted, time specific algorithms to aid providers in deciding fetal heart rate patterns requiring clinical intervention. There is consensus by NICHD that the normal pattern (defined as normal baseline, moderate FHR variability (FHRV), presence of accelerations, and absence of decelerations) confers an extremely high predictability of a normally oxygenated fetus and therefore requires no interventions. At the other end of the spectrum, there is consensus that the pattern of recurrent late or variable decelerations or substantial bradycardia, with absent FHRV, is predictive of current or impending fetal asphyxia so severe that the fetus is at risk of neurologic or other fetal damage or death. In between these 2 extremes are 50% of all other intrapartum fetuses. The need for consensus regarding FHR pattern interpretation and management is particularly important for establishing collaborative practice among physicians, midwives and nurses.[4, 5, 12] **Table 5-1** outlines a three tier FHR interpretation system recommended by the 2008 NICHD Workshop participants.

Providers have traditionally been hesitant to codify guidelines for managing FHR pattern tracings since there is a weak association between variant patterns and significant fetal acidemia and fear exists that written guidelines will be used to scrutinize clinical practice in a court of law. Nonetheless, physicians and midwives have some time frame within which they expect to be notified of specific pattern tracings, and nurses have expectations regarding the speed with which a provider responds to their request for a monitor tracing evaluation. It is also a clinical reality, that practitioners base their interventions on their interpretation of the FHR tracing. In a court proceeding, they will be asked when and by whom they should have been notified, particularly if there was a delay in notification.[4]

The limitations of the EFM do not allow caregivers to know with certainty which fetus is actually hypoxemic or acidemic; thus, all nonreassuring FHR patterns warrant intrauterine resuscitative techniques based on the clinical situation.[13] Intrauterine resuscitative measures in response to a nonreassuring

**Table 5-1  Three-Tier Fetal Heart Rate Interpretation System**

| Category I<br>Normal/includes *all* of the following | Category II<br>Indeterminate/not predictive of abnormal fetal acid-base status, yet cannot be classified as either Category 1 or 11 at this time and include *any* of the following | Category III<br>Abnormal and predictive of abnormal fetal acid-base status at the time of observation<br>Require prompt evaluation and include *either* |
|---|---|---|
| ☐ Baseline rate: 110-160 bpm<br>☐ Moderate baseline variability<br>☐ Absent, late or variable decelerations<br>☐ Present or absent early decelerations<br>☐ Present or absent accelerations | ☐ Bradycardia not accompanied by absent variability<br>☐ Tachycardia<br>☐ Minimal baseline variability<br>☐ Absent baseline variability not accompanied by recurrent decelerations<br>☐ Marked baseline variability<br>☐ Absence of induced accelerations after fetal stimulation<br>☐ Recurrent variable decelerations accompanied by minimal or moderate baseline variability<br>☐ Prolonged deceleration > 2minutes but < 10 minutes<br>☐ Recurrent late decelerations with moderate variability<br>☐ Variable decelerations with other characteristics, such as slow return to baseline, "overshoots", or "shoulders" | ☐ Absent baseline FHR variability and any of the following:<br>  • Recurrent late decelerations<br>  • Recurrent variable decelerations<br>  • Bradycardia<br>☐ Sinusoidal pattern |

Adapted from: Macones G, Hankins G, Spong C, Hauth , Moore T. The 2008 national institute of child health and human development workshop report on electronic fetal monitoring: Update on definitions, interpretation, and research guidelines. Obstetrics & Gynecology 2008; 112: 661-666.

fetal tracing should be second nature to nurses assessing fetal well-being via EFM. The goal is to oxygenate the fetus and includes:

➢ Maternal position change to either left or right side
➢ Increase intravenous fluids
➢ Oxygen via non-rebreather mask at 8-10 liters/min
➢ Discontinue Oxytocin
➢ Tocolytics may be ordered
➢ NOTIFY the provider of your interventions
➢ DOCUMENT all interventions and conversations with the provider

It must also be kept in mind that as labor progresses, the methods used to assess the FHR and uterine activity may change depending on the quality of information received for interpretation and what is needed for adequate assessment, interpretation, clinical interventions and evaluation. **Figure 5-1** depicts AWHONN's Decision Tree for Fetal Heart Monitoring.

---

**Take Home Message**

EFM should be perceived as a screening rather than diagnostic tool. Nurses must always consider electronic indicators within the context of the total clinical picture. At this time, no simple algorithms exist on which to rely and decisions must be made based on critical thinking.

---

**Fetal Monitoring Challenges**
**Multiples**

Multiple gestations can be challenging to monitor and special precautions should be taken to ensure that each fetus is properly assessed. These include:

➢ Each fetus should be identified depending on its location in the abdomen. The fetus that is closest to the maternal cervix is labeled "A" [14]
➢ The position of each fetus in the uterus as well as which fetus corresponds to the dark and light lines on the tracing should also be recorded in the patient record as well as on the tracing [15]
➢ Every effort should be made to keep each labeled fetus on its assigned ultrasound transducer for subsequent monitoring procedures [14]
➢ Always monitor all fetuses at the same time. (As strange as this may seem, I have reviewed medical records in which the physician has ordered that only a particular fetus be monitored.)
➢ Remember to notify the provider if you experience difficulties in obtaining a clear tracing so that other assessment methods may be initiated (i.e., biophysical profile). Also do not forget to DOCUMENT your difficulty, your conversation with the physician or midwife and their follow up!

# Figure 5-1 Decision Tree for Fetal Heart Monitoring

(AWHONN (2003). Fetal Heart Monitoring: Principles & Practice. 3rd ed. Kendall-Hunt. Used with permission.)

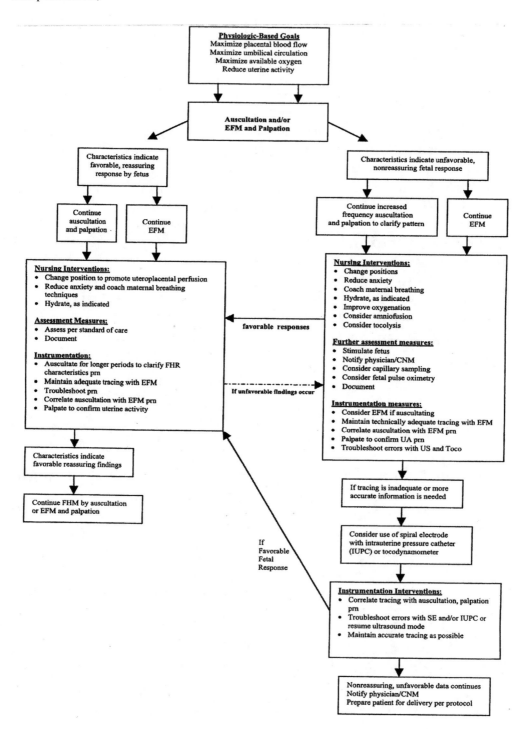

## The Obese Patient

Monitoring of the obese pregnant woman presents many challenges and may require one-to-one care in order for optimum fetal surveillance to be achieved. Induction or augmentation of labor is common in the obese woman due to the increased risk of obstetric complications, such as diabetes and preeclampsia. As with any patient, assessing for hyperstimulation is of utmost importance and obtaining an accurate assessment of uterine activity may be very difficult. Uterine activity typically is monitored with a tocodynamometer, providing frequency and duration of contractions. In obese patients, the distance from the skin to the uterus may be such that the tocodynamometer does not detect contractions reliably and an invasive intrauterine pressure catheter is often required. A fetal scalp electrode may also be necessary should there be difficulty in obtaining a clear tracing of the fetal heart rate that can be easily interpreted.

Providers should be encouraged to alert staff to the anticipated admission of the obese patient well before her due date so that adequate equipment, staffing arrangements and a plan of care can be formulated.

## The Preterm Fetus

The decision of whether to monitor the very preterm fetus is complicated and requires a discussion between the obstetrician, pediatrician, and patient concerning the likelihood of survival. If a patient would undergo a cesarean delivery for fetal indications for a very preterm fetus, monitoring should be achieved continuously rather than intermittently auscultated.[1] Unfortunately, current research has focused on monitoring practices in the term fetus, and there is a clearly identified need for evidence-based research to justify current interpretations regarding the preterm fetus.[16]

Although the principles of EFM are the same for the preterm fetus as the term fetus, there are differences in FHR patterns of preterm fetuses when compared to those in term labor, and there are unique clinical implications for obtaining and interpreting EFM data during preterm labor.[17] In the stabilization period for preterm patients, fetal assessments are completed according to high-risk guidelines outlined by the Association of Women's Health, Obstetrics and Neonatal Nursing (AWHONN) and the American College of Obstetricians and Gynecologists (ACOG).[14, 16, 18, 19] When monitoring the preterm fetus, consideration must also be given to the effect that tocolytics, maternal fever, maternal hydration, or infection may have on the baseline fetal heart rate and variability.[16]

Evidence suggests that nonreassuring FHR patterns have a greater significance for outcomes for the preterm fetus.[20] In preterm infants less than 33 weeks gestation, approximately 70% to 80% of nonreassuring FHR patterns will result in a birth of a neurologically depressed, hypoxemic, or acidemic infant. Also the progression from reassuring to nonreassuring status occurs more often and more quickly in the preterm fetus as compared to the term fetus.[21] Intrauterine resuscitative measures are the same for both the term and preterm fetus.

Even with one-to-one nursing care, in order to obtain a continuous tracing, a very small fetus and/or the presence of multiple fetuses can require frequent adjustments to the fetal monitoring devices. It is important to accurately palpate the uterine fundus and place the external tocodynameter appropriately to detect contractions. Remembering that the fundal height is related to fetal size and gestation age, Leopold maneuvers can assist in determining placement of the external ultrasound device to detect the FHR(s) by identification of the smooth surface of the back of the fetus(es), where the FHR(s) are usually easier to detect. [17]

## Risk Management Strategies in Working with EFM

The electronic fetal monitor is central to most labor and delivery units today. It is also the focal point of many obstetric malpractice cases. In cases in which the obstetrician has been cited for not performing a cesarean delivery in a timely manner, nurses have been seen to contribute to this by failing to interpret the monitor strip and subsequently failing to convey a sense of urgency to the physician.[22] Lack of knowledge, fear of conflict, and poor communication are three areas that contribute to errors especially in EFM interpretation and management.[23] The EFM tracing is also used to correlate the fetal status with the labor progress notes and the testimony of the witnesses.

There are two key components to a successful risk management program: avoiding preventable adverse outcomes and decreasing liability exposure. The former requires competent care providers who speak the same EFM language and who are in a practice environment with systems in place to intervene in a clinically timely manner while the latter includes methods to demonstrate evidence that appropriate, timely care was provided and that fetal status had not deteriorated significantly before the interventions occurred.[24]

Physicians and nurses who institute EFM as an assessment tool of fetal well-being need to possess the knowledge and skills to interpret fetal heart patterns, intervene accordingly and document using approved terminology. The Association of Women's Health, Obstetric and Neonatal Nurses[19] strongly advises that all nurses who perform fetal assessment during the antepartum or intrapartum period complete a course of study that includes the physiologic interpretation of EFM data and its implications for labor support. This course should include instruction in both cognitive and psychomotor skill validations of standardized core competencies used in auscultation, electronic monitoring of the fetal heart rate (FHR) and evaluation of uterine activity. There is no single way of ensuring competency in the interpretation of fetal heart tracings. What is important is that perinatal nurses and providers commit to an educational system or plan that allows them both to update their EFM skills on a regular basis and to stay abreast of the latest technological advances in the field.[22]

The following recommendations can also be beneficial for risk management when EFM is utilized:

➤ Keep in mind that there can be challenges to obtaining interpretable EFM tracings (i.e. obesity, gestational age) and have a plan to assess the fetus with another method should it be necessary.

➤ Be cognizant of the effects medications can have on different fetal heart rate patterns and be able to differentiate what is a normal response from what is an abnormal response to a medication.

➤ All team members should use one common language for FHR patterns for all professional communication and medical record documentation (NICHD terminology)

➤ Adopt the concept that failure to ensure fetal-well being mandates further testing (biophysical profile, scalp pH, or scalp stimulation)[25]

➤ Internal EFM is used if fetal well-being cannot be established either by auscultation or by external monitor.[25]

➤ Establish joint nurse/nurse-midwife/physician EFM educational programs[26] (i.e., Strip reviews, certification )

➤ Print the FHR tracing directly from the fetal monitor and use it to assess fetal status during labor rather than relying solely on the computer screen for ongoing surveillance[26]

➤ Empower nurses to be able to question the interpretation of an EFM strip by another nurse or physician

➤ All nurses should know how and when to initiate intrauterine resuscitative measures

➤ In women requiring cesarean delivery, fetal surveillance should continue until the abdominal sterile preparation has begun. If internal fetal heart rate monitoring is in use, it should be continued until the abdominal sterile prep is completed.[27]

➤ Conduct medical record audits which provide substantial data about the requisite knowledge base and essential clinical skills during the intrapartum period[24]

➤ All nurses should be familiar with the Chain of Command policy and how to activate it if a conflict should arise

➤ Each health care facility should develop a policy that defines when it is appropriate to use auscultation and when to use EFM. It should specify the frequency of assessment and documentation for each methodology. The institutional protocol for frequency of FHR auscultation should incorporate the best available evidence, professional association guidelines and practitioner expert consensus.[19]

> Institutions can develop guidelines that include: FHR patterns that will trigger midwife or physician notification; time frames within which notification should be accomplished; which patterns require midwife and/or physician bedside evaluation [4]

> Treat the fetal monitor tracing as a legal document - follow hospital policy on the maintenance and storage of fetal monitor strips. Requirements for record retention vary by state, but because EFM tracings may be sought as evidence long after the plaintiff's date of birth, a long term storage policy is advised. If those records cannot be produced, the defense faces a serious challenge. Plaintiffs may raise the question of purposeful destruction of evidence, and jurors are left to question if poor record keeping is a sign of broader negligence.[28]

> The best time to review your institution's EFM tracing retention policy is before you need to rely upon it. Take time now to review your policy and procedures, especially if such review has not been recently performed. A single runaway jury award in an obstetric-related malpractice case can devastate individual providers and tarnish a hospital's image. Hazarding such outcomes due to inadequate record retention is an unnecessary risk.[28]

## Documentation

Documentation (of both oral and written communication) should always be viewed as an essential element in the care of the laboring patient and a venue for maintaining cohesiveness among health team members. Accurate timing and description of intrapartal events in chronological order cannot be overemphasized.[29] (From 2003-2007, issues related to documentation of labor and delivery were a factor in 17 claims or suits filed against the insurer of the Harvard affiliated hospitals in Massachusetts. This represented 27.8 million dollars. In some cases, the defense had to contend with the fact that the EFM strips could not be located and produced for trial.) National guidelines for documentation of regular assessments of the strip chart include using specific, recognized nomenclature to identify the FHR pattern. This means using terms such as "late deceleration" or "variable deceleration" both in verbal and written communication.[14]

In the case of a nonreassuring FHR of acute onset resulting in an emergent cesarean birth, summary documentation should include but not be limited to the following[14]:

> Time the nonreassuring fetal heart rate was recognized
> Nursing actions initiated for maternal and/or fetal resuscitation
> Continued FHR assessment to evaluate the fetal response to interventions
> Communication with the team members and their responses
> Time the woman was taken to the operating room and time of incision
> Chronologies of interventions performed and by whom for newborn resuscitation if necessary
> A narrative note reflecting discussion between health care providers and the woman and her family

Documentation of the time of events and the results of intrauterine resuscitative interventions in response to nonreassuring patterns are of paramount importance since minutes can mean the difference between a good or a poor outcome. Should litigation ensue and years have passed, it is virtually impossible to reenact particular aspects of an event without having some frame of reference. Plaintiff attorneys rely on this to enhance their case in the eyes of the jury. After all, it is difficult to fathom how the average intrapartal nurse could remember whether he/she recognized the nonreassuring fetal status, performed certain interventions, assessed the effectiveness of the interventions and notified the provider with a timely response resulting.[29]

The terms "fetal distress" and "birth asphyxia" should not be used per ACOG's Committee on Obstetric Practice.[30] These terms are imprecise and nonspecific. The term, "fetal distress," has a low positive predictive value even in high-risk populations and often is associated with an infant who is in good condition at birth as determined by the Apgar score or umbilical cord blood gas analysis or both. The communication between clinicians caring for the woman and those caring for her neonate is best served by replacing the term fetal distress with "nonreassuring fetal status," followed by a further description of findings (e.g., repetitive variable decelerations, fetal tachycardia or bradycardia, late decelerations, or low biophysical profile).

During emergent intrapartum situations, some nurses feel that documentation directly on the fetal monitoring tracing can assist them in constructing notes after patient stabilization. If this approach is used, it is important to ensure that the content and times included in the narrative coincide with the fetal monitoring tracing annotations.[14] While notations directly on the FHR tracing can be useful during emergent situations, the practice of duplicate documentation of routine care on both the FHR tracing and the medical record is no longer recommended.[31] Hand writing on the tracing about routine care not only can decrease the amount of nursing time spent on patient care activities, but this practice also can lead to errors in documentation and can contribute to delays in transcription to the medical record.[32]

---

**Take Home Message**

EFM as a stand-alone tool is ineffective in avoiding preventable adverse outcomes. It is effective only when used in accordance with published standards and guidelines by professionals skilled in correct interpretation and when appropriate timely intervention is based on that interpretation. Interpretation and intervention are best accomplished as a collaborative perinatal team rather than an individual activity.[6]

---

**Did You Know?**

For the neonate who is suspected of having undergone a severe asphyxial episode at some time during gestation, several blood tests may assist in the determination of when and how the episode occurred. The cord blood provides valuable data with the arterial pH, nucleated red blood cells (NRBCs), and platelet levels. The NRBC count, SGOT, SGPT, serum creatinine, and serum sodium levels should be monitored for several days. In the context of the prenatal and intrapartum history and the clinical condition of the neonate, these hematologic markers may provide physicians with information regarding the timing and severity of the fetal asphyxial insult.[33]

The placenta may also offer clues to the timing and occurrence of antenatal events should there be an adverse outcome. If there is a medical malpractice suit filed, a placental defense can become instrumental in winning the case. It is imperative that the placenta be properly identified and the appropriate paperwork accompany it to pathology.[34]

---

1. ACOG Practice Bulletin. Intrapartum fetal heart rate monitoring. Washington, DC: ACOG; 2005; 70.

2. Parer JT. Electronic fetal heart rate monitoring: A story of survival. *Obstet Gynecol Surv.* 2003; 58:561-563.

3. Clark SL, Hankins GD. Temporal and demographic trends in cerebral palsy: Fact and fiction. *American Journal of Obstetrics & Gynecology.* 2003; 188:628-633.

4. Fox M, Kilpatrick S, King T, Parer JT. Fetal heart rate monitoring: Interpretation and collaborative management. *J Midwifery Womens Health.* 2000; 45:498-507.

5. The National Institute of Child Health and Human Development Research Planning Workshop. Electronic fetal heart rate monitoring: Research guidelines for interpretation. *JOGNN.* 1997: 635-640.

6. Simpson KR. Perinatal patient safety. Standardized language for electronic fetal heart rate monitoring. *MCN.* 2004; 29:336.

7. Gilbert E. *Manual of High Risk Pregnancy & Delivery.* 4th ed. St. Louis, Missouri: Mosby; 2007.

8. Rostant D, Cady R. *Liability Issues in Perinatal Nursing.* Philadelphia: Lippincott; 1999.

9. Dwyer M. EFM expertise. *Forum.* 2007; 25:6-7.

10. Miller LA. Finally, consensus!. *J Perinat Neonatal Nurs.* 2005; 19:291-292.

11. Cherouny PH, Federico FA, Haraden C, Leavitt Gullo S, Resar R. Idealized design of perinatal care. IHI innovation series white paper. Cambridge, Massachusetts: Institution for Healthcare Improvement; 2005. Available from: www.IHI.org.

12. Parer JT, Ikeda T. A framework for standardized management of intrapartum fetal heart rate patterns. *Am J Obstet Gynecol.* 2007; 197:26.e1-26.e6.

13. Simpson KR. Failure to rescue: Implications for evaluating quality of care during labor and birth. *J Perinat Neonat Nurs.* 2005; 19:24-36.

14. Feinstein N, Torgersen K, Atterbury J, eds. *Fetal Heart Monitoring Principles and Practice.* 3rd ed. Dubuque, Iowa: Kendall/Hunt; 2003.

15. Murray M. *Antepartal and Intrapartal Fetal Monitoring.* 2nd ed. New York: Springer; 1997.

16. Baird S, Ruth D. Electronic fetal monitoring of the preterm fetus. *The Journal of Perinatal and Neonatal Nursing.* 2002; 16:12-24.

17. Simpson KR. Monitoring the preterm fetus during labor. *MCN Am J Matern Child Nurs.* 2004; 29:380-388.

18. ACOG Practice Bulletin. Assessment of risk factors for preterm birth. Washington, DC: ACOG; 2001; 31.

19. AWHONN. Clinical position statement on fetal assessment. Washington, DC: AWHONN; 2002.

20. Matsuda Y, Maeda T, Kouno S. The critical period of non-reassuring fetal heart rate patterns in preterm gestation. *Eur J Obstet Gynecol Reprod Biol.* 2003; 106:36-39.

21. Freeman RK, Garite TJ, Nageotte M. *Fetal Heart Rate Monitoring.* 3rd ed. Philadelphia: Lippincott,Williams & Wilkins; 2003.

22. Greenwald LM, Mondor M. Malpractice and the perinatal nurse. *J Perinat Neonat Nurs.* 2003; 17:101-109.

23. Miller LA. System errors in intrapartum electronic fetal monitoring: A case review. *J Midwifery Womens Health.* 2005; 50:507-516.

24. Simpson KR, Knox EG. Risk management and electronic fetal monitoring: Decreasing risk of adverse outcomes and liability exposure. *J Perinat Neonat Nurs.* 2000; 14:40-52.

25. Knox GE, Simpson K. High reliability perinatal units: An approach to the prevention of patient injury and medical malpractice claims. *Journal of Healthcare Risk Management.* 1999; 19:24-32.

26. Simpson KR, Knox GE. Common areas of litigation related to care during labor and birth: Recommendations to promote patient safety and decrease risk exposure. *J Perinat Neonat Nurs.* 2003; 17:110-127.

27. American Academy of of Pediatrics (AAP) and American College of Obstetricians and Gynecologists (ACOG). *Guidelines for Perinatal Care.* 5th ed. Washington, DC: Author; 2002.

28. Strategies for patient safety. 2008. Available from: www.crico/rmf@rmf. harvard.edu. Accessed March 3, 2008.

29. Connors P. High -risk perinatal issues:Delay in the diagnosis of fetal distress and insufficient documentaion. *Journal of Nursing Law.* 2003; 9:19-26.

30. American College of Obstetricians and Gynecologists Committee on Obstetric Practice. Inappropriate use of the terms fetal distress and birth asphyxia. Washington DC: American College of Obstetricians and Gynecologists; 2005; 326:1469-1470.

31. Simpson K, Creehan P. *Perinatal Nursing.* 3rd ed. Philadelphia: Lippincott Williams & Wilkins:; 2008.

32. Chez BF. Electronic fetal monitoring: Then and now. *Journal of Perinatal and Neonatal Nursing.* 1997; 10:1-4.

33. Phelan JP, Martin GI, Korst LM. Birth asphyxia and cerebral palsy. *Clinics in Perinatology.* 2005; 32:61-76.

34. American Society for Healthcare Risk Management Obstetrics Task Force, ed. *Risk Management Pearls for Obstetrics.* Chicago, IL: American Hospital Association; 2000.

# CHAPTER 6

# OB Drugs
# That Demand Respect

When researchers analyzed data about perinatal medication errors reported to the United States Pharmacopeia MEDMARX program, they found that more than 300 medications were named in reports to MEDMARX about medication errors in labor and delivery units, obstetric recovery rooms, and postpartum maternity units. Nurse distractions and workload increases were the most commonly reported factors contributing to error.[1] Magnesium sulfate, Oxytocin, insulin, (all of which are on the Institute for Safe Medication's High Alert Medication List) and antibiotics, such as ampicillin and penicillin G, were named the most often. Errors involving these medications have resulted in severe complications and even death. Though we do not use the quantity of medications our med-surg colleagues do, we should never underestimate the potency of these medications or feel immune to the possibility of a patient being harmed.

Tragic cases such as the one reported in Wisconsin in which an experienced nurse, working a double shift, mistakenly administered a bag of epidural anesthesia (instead of penicillin) intravenously, causing the death of her 16-year-old patient and the death of 3 preterm infants in Indiana from overdoses of heparin, are truly wake up calls to the need for vigilance and safety in medication administration. In the Wisconsin case, the nurse was cited for not following the five rights of medication administration and was threatened with 6 years of incarceration and a fine of $25,000. (www.wha.org/legalAndRegulatory/DOJcriminalcomplaint 11-2-06.pdf) After plea bargaining, the nurse was placed on 3 years probation, received a suspension of her nursing license for 9 months, and is prohibited from working long hours for at least 2 years.[2]

**Cervical Ripening Agents**

*Because of the lack of knowledge about the exact physiology of labor, it is difficult to determine the optimal dosages necessary to correct abnormal labor with artificial pharmalogic compounds. Consequently hyperstimulation may occur during cervical ripening and induction or augmentation of labor with Oxytocin or other prostaglandin compounds. Each woman has an individual myometrial sensitivity to Oxytocin and prostaglandin.[3]*

There are several methods available for ripening the cervix that are not favorable for induction. Regardless of the method used, the nurse must be aware of the risks, benefits, and limitations of the method selected. There may also be a fine line between cervical ripening and the actual induction of labor. The nurse caring for the patient must be vigilant for assessing for the onset of labor. There is a lack of data about the type and intensity of maternal-fetal assessments for women undergoing cervical ripening. Monitoring of the patient should be individualized by taking into consideration maternal-fetal status before administration of the drug, the maternal-fetal response to the drug, and the indications for cervical ripening and induction as well as the pharmacokinetics of the drug. Development of institutional guidelines and protocols for each pharmacologic agent, based on review of available data and consensus among perinatal nurses, obstetricians, and nurse midwives, is essential to provide a foundation of safe and effective clinical care.[4]

## Misoprostol (Cytotec)

Misoprostol is a synthetic analogue of naturally occurring prostaglandin-E1 used in the treatment and prevention of gastric ulcers caused by non-steroidal anti-inflammatory drugs. Currently it is not approved by the U.S. Food and Drug Administration for cervical ripening or induction of labor. However, it is widely used and has proven to be very effective in both cervical ripening and induction of labor. Misoprostol appears to be a safe and efficient agent when used in the lowest dose needed to achieve desired outcomes.[5] If Misoprostol is used for cervical ripening and induction, one quarter of a 100-ug tablet should be considered an initial dose. Doses should not be administered more frequently than every 3-6 hours and Oxytocin should not be administered less than 4 hours after the last Misoprostol dose. It is not recommended for use in patients with prior cesarean delivery or major uterine surgery.[6]

Misoprostol can be administered by perinatal nurses; however, in many institutions, this practice is deferred to physicians and midwives. If Misoprostol administration is delegated to perinatal nurses, they must have demonstrated competence in insertion, and the activity must be within the scope of practice as defined by state and provincial regulations.[7]

## Cervidil

Cervidil vaginal insert is easily inserted into the fornix of the vagina and works by releasing Dinoprostone upon absorbing moisture. It is removed after 12 hours or when active labor begins.[8] One advantage of Cervidil is that the system can be easily and quickly removed in the event of uterine hyperstimulation or complications. If uterine hyperstimulation occurs, complete reversal of the prostaglandin–induced uterine pattern usually occurs within 15 minutes of removal. If necessary, the woman may be given tocolytic therapy (0.25 mg of Terbutaline subcutaneously).

**Oxytocin (Pitocin)**

Oxytocin is recognized and respected as potentially the most dangerous drug used in obstetrics and the most preventable cause of perinatal liability.[9] In successful malpractice claims, a common recurring problem is the inappropriate use of Oxytocin leading to uterine hyperstimulation, uterine rupture, nonreassuring fetal status, depressed newborns at birth, long term neurologic sequelae and/ or fetal death.[9] Common allegations that are made when Oxytocin is used for induction or augmentation include:[10]

  ➤ Failure to fully inform the woman of the risks and benefits of elective induction
  ➤ Failure to accurately determine gestational age prior to induction
  ➤ Iatrogenic prematurity as a result of elective induction before 39 completed weeks of pregnancy
  ➤ Excessive doses of Oxytocin resulting in hyperstimulation of uterine activity (with or without the presence of a non reassuring FHR pattern)
  ➤ Failure to accurately assess maternal-fetal status during labor induction

Oxytocin is used to both induce labor and to augment ineffective contractions in terms of strength or frequency so that labor may progress. Critical elements that must be considered when Oxytocin is used include:[8, 11]

  ➤ Assessment of gestational age-before the elective induction of labor is initiated, it must be determined that the fetus has a gestational age of 39 weeks, and this determination must be documented according to agreed upon standards. (ACOG guidelines[8] and other research report that the likelihood of harm to the baby from elective induction is greater before 39 weeks. In the event of an adverse outcome, plaintiffs' attorneys may use non-compliance with this guideline as an indicator of poor care).
  ➤ Estimated fetal weight. It is important to know the size of the fetus to determine whether a continued attempt at vaginal delivery is appropriate if augmentation is initiated.
  ➤ Informed consent including risk and benefits, reason for induction, agents and methods of labor induction and possible need for a repeat induction or cesarean section
  ➤ Availability of a physician capable of performing a cesarean section.
  ➤ Electronic monitoring of the fetal heart rate for reassurance. Clinicians monitor the fetal heart rate and the effects of uterine stimulants on the fetus. A standard definition of *reassurance* needs to be understood by all team members. Use of the NICHD fetal monitoring terminology as accepted by both ACOG and AWHONN ensures this.
  ➤ Pelvic assessment - to determine dilation, effacement, station, cervical position and consistency (Bishop's score) and fetal presentation should

be performed and documented before the induction is initiated.

➤ Monitoring and management of hyperstimulation. *Hyperstimulation* is a series of single contractions lasting 2 minutes or more, contractions of normal duration occurring within 1 minute of each other or a contraction frequency of five or more in 10 minutes[7, 8] Some authors reserve the term *hyperstimulation* for a contraction frequency of more than five in 10 minutes with evidence that the fetus is not tolerating this labor pattern as evidenced by late decelerations or bradycardia. Definitions of *hyperstimulation* that include evidence of nonreassuring fetal status are not clinically appropriate because such definitions may delay interventions to reduce uterine activity while fetal status deteriorates.[12] A clear definition of *hyperstimulation* needs to be agreed upon by team members because clinical management strategies, policies, and protocols should include what actions are expected when hyperstimulation is identified.[12] It should also be noted that the term tachysystole applies to both spontaneous or stimulated labor and is the preferred term of ACOG.[13]

To minimize the opportunity for harm, it is necessary to understand the pharmacology of the drug and its impact on the fetus, and to have protocols to guide its appropriate use.[11] Each hospital's department of obstetrics and gynecology should develop written protocols for preparing and administering Oxytocin for labor induction or augmentation. Indications for induction or augmentation should be stated as well as the qualifications of personnel authorized to administer oxytocic agents.[6]

Oxytocin can be administered orally, nasally, intramuscularly or intravenously. Buccal, nasal, or intramuscular administration of Oxytocin should not be used to induce or augment labor.[6] The intravenous route is used to stimulate the pregnant uterus because it allows precise measurement of the amount of medication being administered and a relatively rapid discontinuation of the drug when side effects occur.[14] When administered intravenously, Oxytocin is piggybacked into the mainline solution at the port most proximal to the venous site. There are many variations in the dilution rate. Some protocols suggest adding 10 units of Oxytocin to 1,000 mL of an isotonic electrolyte solution, resulting in an infusion dosage rate of 1 mU/min=6mL/h. However, other commonly reported dilutions are 20 units in 1,000 mL IV fluid (1 mU/min=3mL/h) and 60 units of Oxytocin to 1,000 IV fluid (1mU/min=1mL/h). There are no clear advantages for any one dilution rate. The key issues are knowledge of how many milliunits per minute are administered and consistency in clinical practice within each institution. To enhance communication among members of the perinatal health care team and to avoid confusion, Oxytocin administration rates should always be ordered by the physician or CNM as milliunits per minute and documented in the medical record as milliunits per minute.[7, 8]

**Nursing Responsibilities**

The nurse administering Oxytocin, whether it is for augmentation or induction, must have a clear understanding of her duties and responsibilities. These include:

> Knowledge of the pharmacodynamics and pharmacokinetics of Oxytocin

> Awareness of 1:2 nurse-to-patient ratio.[6] If a nurse cannot clinically evaluate the effects of medication at least every 15 minutes, the Oxytocin infusion should not be started or needs to be terminated if infusing.[8]

> Understanding of the labor process including uterine contraction physiology and endogenous Oxytocin secretion

> Knowledge of the reason for induction

> Delaying starting the administration of Oxytocin if the patient expresses inadequate knowledge of the procedure including risks and benefits and notifies the provider of her observations

> Understanding the definition, physiology and effects of hyperstimulation on the fetus and laboring woman

> Knowledge and understanding of the titration process in response to fetal-maternal response. The titration process includes decreasing the dosage rate when contractions are too frequent or fetal status is nonreassuring and increasing the dosage rate when uterine activity and progress of labor slows.[14, 15]

> Knowledge of the hospital's policy for Oxytocin administration

> Knowledge of intrauterine resuscitative measures

> Knowledge of the Chain of Command policy and a commitment to follow it if necessary[15]

> Appreciation of ongoing education of standards to guide their practice[15]

> Remembering that if labor is progressing within normal limits, there is no need to increase the administration rate.[7]

Nurses must also be cognizant that, while physician's orders are written in the chart and establish the parameters of Oxytocin administration, it is the nurse's responsibility to titrate the Oxytocin based on the frequency of uterine contractions, the progress of labor, and fetal tolerance. This is true no matter what induction/augmentation protocol is used. The nurse's decision-making process is critical because an inappropriate decision regarding how to manage Oxytocin may lead to fetal compromise.[15] **Table 6-1** is a suggested clinical protocol addressing oxytocin induced uterine tachysystole. Most fetuses enter labor with large reserve of placental capacity that helps to accommodate the repeated

**Table 6-1  Suggested Clinical Protocol for Oxytocin Induced Uterine Tachysystole**

| Reassuring (Normal) FHR | Nonreassuring FHR | Resumption of Oxytocin After Resolution of Hyperstimulation |
|---|---|---|
| • Maternal repositioning.<br>• IV fluid bolus of approximately 500 mL of Lactated Ringer's solution.<br>• If uterine activity has not returned to normal after 10 minutes, decrease Oxytocin rate at least half; if uterine activity is less than 5 contractions in 10 minutes.<br>• NOTIFY the provider. | • Discontinue Oxytocin.<br>• Maternal repositioning.<br>• IV fluid bolus of approximately 500 mL of Lactated Ringer's solution.<br>• Consider oxygen at 10 L/min via non-rebreather facemask if the first interventions mentioned previously do not resolve the nonreassuring (indeterminate or abnormal) FHR pattern; discontinue as soon as possible<br>• If no response, consider 0.25 mg terbutaline subcutaneously<br>• NOTIFY primary provider of actions taken and maternal-fetal response. | • If Oxytocin has been discontinued for less than 20-30 minutes, the FHR is reassuring, and contraction frequency, intensity, and duration are normal, resume Oxytocin at no more than half the rate that caused the tachysystole and gradually increase the rate needed as appropriate based on unit protocol and maternal-fetal status.<br>• If Oxytocin is discontinued for more than 30-40 minutes, resume Oxytocin at initial dose ordered. |

Reference: Simpson, K. & Knox, E. (2009). Oxytocin as a high alert medication: Implications for perinatal patient safety. *MCN: The American Journal of Maternal-Child Nursing*, 34 (1). Copyright 2009 by Lippincott Williams & Wilkins. Reprinted with permission.

brief reductions in oxygen during contractions. The effects of repeated hypoxia may be amplified in vulnerable fetuses (i.e., fetuses with preexisting placental insufficiency). Conversely, even a normal fetus with normal placental function may be unable to adapt fully to tonic contractions or uterine hyperstimulation.[16] A bedside evaluation by the attending physician is needed to increase beyond 20 mU/minute. This should be considered only in unusual clinical situations.[12]

If a clinical disagreement ensues between the provider's order and your nursing judgment about the intervention for the patient, it may be helpful to review your professional organization's standards and hospital policies with the provider.[15] If this does not resolve the issue, you must choose to talk with the charge nurse, and institute the chain of command if necessary.

### Assessment and Documentation

When EFM is used to record FHR data permanently, periodic documentation can be used to summarize fetal status as outlined by institutional protocols. During Oxytocin induction or augmentation, at a minimum, the FHR should be documented before every dosage increase. If the dosage is maintained at the same rate, a reasonable approach is for nurses to document the FHR at least every hour during Oxytocin administration.[7] Uterine contractions should be assessed with every dosage increase and if it is maintained at the same rate, a reasonable approach is for nurses to document uterine activity at least every hour.[7] Assessment should be done by palpation, tocodynamometer, or an intrauterine pressure catheter. The uterine frequency, duration, intensity and relaxation between contractions must be addressed. (Do not confuse this with the need for evaluating and assessing the FHR every 15 minutes in the first stage of labor and every 5 minutes during the second stage.[6])

### Complications Follow Questionable Induction of Labor[17]

A healthy 30-year-old, G 4 P 2, entered Labor and Delivery for induction at 40 weeks. The patient had a Mc Donald's cerclage at 14 weeks gestation which was removed by her obstetrician at 36 weeks. Her cervix was notable for a laceration and scarring at the 4 o'clock position. Her obstetrician scheduled an induction of labor (the indication was not documented). Examination in Labor and Delivery revealed that her cervix was 1 cm dilated. Pitocin was ordered to induce labor, and the obstetrician attempted to rupture the amniotic membranes on three separate occasions over six hours without success. The fetal heart rate tracing (FHR) was reactive throughout the day. Pitocin was stopped in the late afternoon because the patient's cervix did not dilate. She was sent home with plans to return in a few days.

Six days later, the patient returned for a second induction.

| | |
|---|---|
| 9:00 a.m. | The patient's cervix was 1-2 cm. and long, and the FHR had mild-moderate variability with the baseline of 140-150 beats per minute (bpm). Prostin gel was placed to ripen the cervix and Pitocin started "per protocol." |
| 12:30 p.m. | Her cervix was 2-3 cm dilated and the FHR tracing had moderate variability with occasional variable decelerations. |
| 1:30 p.m. | She received an epidural for pain relief, and her cervix was about 4 cm dilated. Her amniotic fluid sac ruptured spontaneously and a "small amount, blood-tinged" fluid was noted. |
| 3:00 p.m. | Her cervix was 5 cm dilated, the FHR was 140 bpm with minimal variability and variable decelerations around the time of contractions. |
| 7:00 p.m. | The patient's cervix was 8 cm dilated and the fetal head at 1+/2+ station. The FHR was 160-170 bpm with minimal variability and variable decelerations, some with slow return to baseline. The patient complained of left-sided pain and her epidural was reinforced. |
| 7:30 p.m. | Cervix was an anterior lip. The FHR was 170 bpm with persistent variable decelerations. |
| 9:00 p.m. | The FHR baseline was 170 bpm with deep decelerations. An intrauterine pressure catheter was used to record contractions. The patient complained of severe pain and a fetal scalp electrode was applied. |
| 9:35 p.m. | No cervical change. The FHR was 170 bpm with deep decelerations. The obstetricians decided to deliver by cesarean section. A female infant was found free-floating in the abdomen, requiring resuscitation. The mother's uterus and bladder had ruptured. The infant was severely asphyxiated with extensive neurologic injury, and died three weeks later. |

The parents sued the obstetrician and the case settled in the high range (>$500,000).

**Analysis**

1. The indication for inducing labor prior to the patient's due date, especially with an unripe cervix, was unclear and undocumented.

   *A pregnant woman should be counseled regarding potential risks to her and her fetus, agents and methods of labor stimulation, and the possible need for a repeat induction or a cesarean section instead of a vaginal delivery. The rational for the procedure or treatment, risks involved, expected benefits, and alternatives to treatment including the likely results of no treatment should be documented in the patient's medical record.*

2. The obstetrician failed to recognize that the fetal heart tracing deteriorated during the course of labor, reflecting worsening fetal status and fetal acidosis.

   *Per the American College of Obstetrics and Gynecology, FHR tracings that begin with moderate variability, progressing to minimal or no variability with persistent deepening decelerations are indicative of deteriorating fetal status and require evaluation for possible causes.*

3. Several factors likely contributed to the uterine rupture during labor, including the lacerated and scarred cervix that prevented normal dilation in response to labor contractions, and the integrity of cervical tissue at the laceration site.

   *A scheduled induction should have given the care team maximum opportunity to review the chart and be alert for such risks, circumstances that could be highlighted in a Labor and Delivery team briefing. A huddle or checklist review of concerns prior to the induction of labor and repeated intrapartum as the need arises can help raise the appropriate red flags and increase situational awareness.*

4. The patient alleged that the standard of care was breached when the obstetrician failed to recognize deteriorating fetal status and failed to perform a cesarean section in a timely fashion. The obstetrician could not explain why he did not respond to the deteriorating FHR pattern, and the nurse in this delivery did not convey her concerns about the FHR tracings.

   *Effective communication and teamwork skills might have facilitated the nurse's ability to speak up and discuss her concerns, and enhanced the obstetrician's awareness of the gravity of the situation.*

5. The patient argued that substandard care during the course of labor and delivery led to her daughter's demise.

   *Experts who reviewed the case for the defense concluded that earlier detection of deteriorating fetal status, and earlier intervention, would likely have averted the infant death.*

## Magnesium Sulfate

Magnesium sulfate, which is used to treat both preterm labor and preeclampsia, has been involved in many errors, some of which have been fatal. Most of these errors were due to unfamiliarity with safe dosage ranges and signs of toxicity, inadequate patient monitoring, pump programming errors, and mix ups between magnesium sulfate and Oxytocin.[18] Deaths in seven cases reported by Knox and Simpson[19] were seen to be related to patient transfers to units with lower staffing levels and chaotic environments with changing nursing assignments.

Due to the serious risk of causing significant patient harm, magnesium sulfate is on the Institute of Safe Medication Practices "List of High-Alert Medications."

---

**Examples of Magnesium Sulfate Errors Reported by Simpson and Knox[19]**

#1      A nurse prepared a bag of magnesium sulfate (40g/L) and began an infusion at 200 mL/hour to deliver a 4 g bolus dose (100mL) over 30 minutes. After remaining with the patient for 20 minutes, the nurse was suddenly called away for an urgent problem. She returned 25 minutes later to find the patient had received a 6 g loading dose. The patient was flushed and nauseated, with shallow respirations and unable to move her extremities. Concerned about toxicity, the physician ordered a test of the solution, which revealed a concentration of 80 g/L. The nurse had misread the vial labels and added too much magnesium sulfate to the bag. The patient actually received a 12 g loading dose but subsequently recovered without permanent harm.

#2      A nurse accidentally restarted an infusion of magnesium sulfate instead of beginning a new infusion of Oxytocin after a mother had delivered her baby. The magnesium sulfate infusion had been administered during preterm labor, but it remained connected to the Y-site to the patient although it had been discontinued and was no longer infusing. The Oxytocin solution was connected to the patient, but the magnesium sulfate solution was actually started by mistake. The mother was found unresponsive and remains in a vegetative state.

---

**Safe Care Practices for the Use of Magnesium Sulfate**
      The following are Safe Care Practices for the Use of Magnesium Sulfate in Obstetrics[20]
- Unit policies, protocols, and standing orders should be consistent with what is taught to all healthcare providers. Individual orders from each physician should be avoided.
- Magnesium sulfate should never be abbreviated.
- The pharmacy should supply high-risk IV medications in premixed solutions.
- Use a 100-mL (4g) or 150-mL (6g) IVPB solution for the initial bolus instead of blousing from the main bag with a rate change on the pump.
- Use 500-mL IV bags with 20 g of magnesium sulfate versus 1000-mL IV bags with 40 g of magnesium sulfate for the maintenance fluids.

- Use color-coded tags on the lines as they go into the pumps and into the IV ports.
- Provide 1:1 nursing care at the bedside during the first hour of administration.
- Provide 1:2-3 nursing care during the maintenance dose in a clinical setting in which the patient is close to the nurses' station rather than on the general antepartum or postpartum nursing unit, where nurses are responsible for more patients.
- Consider that a woman receiving magnesium sulfate remains high-risk even when symptoms of pre-eclampsia or preterm are stable.
- Have a second nurse double-check all doses and pump settings.
- When care is transferred to another nurse, have both nurses together at the bedside assess the patient status, review dosage and pump settings, and review written physician medication orders.
- Discontinue the medication once it is completed by removing the line from the IV port.
- Implement periodic magnesium sulfate overdose drills with airway management and calcium administration, with physician and nurse team members participating together.
- Maintain calcium antidote in an easily accessible locked medication kit with the dosage clearly printed on the top.

**Risk Management Strategies for Medication Administration**

Medication errors are the most common, and potentially dangerous, of nursing errors. The following suggestions are made to help you avoid harming your patient and having to live with the psychological trauma of having done so:

- *Always* follow the 5 rights of safe medication administration - right patient, right dose, right medication, right route and right time
- Double check all medication calculations and fluid rates.
- Do not hesitate to ask a colleague to check your calculations.
- Never administer a medication a colleague has prepared.
- If a colleague does ask you to medicate his/her patient, always remember to check the administration record and follow the five rights of medication administration.
- Barcode technology allows rapid processing of information to achieve the "five rights" of the medication process and has been reported to decrease administration errors by 80%.[21]
- On admission, ask patients specifically about prescription medication, over-the-counter (OTC) medication, and herbal remedies being taken.[22 P-47]

- Reconcile all medications and update during the patient's hospitalization.
- When administering blood products, follow facility policies and procedures, for administering, charting and monitoring.[22 P-47]
- Know how to use administration equipment such as pumps and if you are not familiar with them, ask to have an in-service.
- Limit the number of different kinds of infusion devices.[23]
- Keep current on medications that are used in your unit (i.e. the use of high versus low dose Oxytocin).
- Complete a Safety Report (Incident Report) should an error occur.
- Report all pharmacy errors as they are not immune to making mistakes and are striving to improve patient safety just as all members of the team are.
- Avoid cluttered, poorly lit, noisy work spaces when preparing medications.
- Avoid rushing or being constantly interrupted when preparing a medication.
- Remember that as a nurse you are responsible for questioning any medication order that is not within the normal range for dosage or administration route, or is contraindicated due to allergies or medical problems.[24 P-32] Follow these suggestions should you question a medication order:
  - ❖ Refer to a reliable drug reference. Your hospital should make this resource readily available to you and if one is not available, request that your unit receive one immediately.
  - ❖ Call the pharmacist and explain your concern.
  - ❖ Contact the prescribing physician/CNM/Nurse Practitioner and be clear and assertive in questioning the order.
  - ❖ Consult with your charge nurse or supervisor.
  - ❖ Initiate the Chain of Command if necessary.
  - ❖ Remember that you have the legal right not to administer a drug that you feel may harm the patient. You must remember if you choose to do this that: 1) your immediate supervisor and the provider must be notified and 2) document that the drug was not given and why.[22]

The Massachusetts Nurses Association has also addressed the essential environmental conditions conducive to safe medication practices in the "Nurses' Six Rights for Safe Medication Administration" which is available on http:// www.massnurses.org/nurse_practice/sixrights.htm.

The six rights include the:
1. *Right* to a complete and clearly written order.
2. *Right* to have the correct route and dose dispensed.
3. *Right* to have access to information.
4. *Right* to have policies on administration.
5. *Right* to administer medications safely and to identify problems in the system.
6. *Right* to stop, think, and be vigilant when administering medications.

---

**Examples of Medication Errors from Around the Country - personal experiences seminar attendees have shared with me.**

An attendee's sister-in-law was pregnant with twins at 28 weeks when she was admitted to the hospital in preterm labor. Instead of receiving magnesium sulfate, she was given Pitocin and went into labor. Neither twin survived.

The sister of another attendee also was admitted in preterm labor with twins. She was 32 weeks Again, Pitocin was hung instead of magnesium sulfate. She delivered her twins who did survive but spent 5 months in the NICU.

An RN noticed that the Pitocin she was about to administer to her patient had been mixed in *Mannitol* by the pharmacy.

A physician attending an EFM course I was teaching shared with the group that when she was a resident, a student nurse removed her patient's IVs from the pump to facilitate her ambulating to the bathroom. The patient received a bolus of magnesium sulfate and subsequently died.

In responding to the alarms on her patient's pump, a nurse found the patient's husband, a paramedic, pushing buttons on the magnesium sulfate pump in an attempt to silence the alarm. He wanted to be "helpful."

After delivering her patient, a CNM noted that her patent's flow was excessive and, despite her attempts at massage, was having difficulty getting the uterus to contract. She looked up to find that the nurse assisting her had mistakenly removed the Pitocin used for induction and was running in the magnesium sulfate, which the patient had also been receiving, at a bolus rate.

---

**Did You Know?**

#1      Stock-piling drugs in patient areas is risky for two reasons. First, bypassing the pharmacy dispensing system prevents the pharmacy from screening orders and detecting drug interactions, excessive dosages, and little-known cross-allergies to specific drugs. Second, using stock drugs eliminates the important double-check feature of a unit dose dispensing system. As a result, staff may have to calculate, draw up, and mix doses from bulk supplies or unit stock, and these policies set the stage for error.[25]

#2      According to studies, most patients who developed liver toxicity while taking acetaminophen received more than 4 g daily. Healthcare providers need to keep track of patient's total daily doses to make sure they do not exceed safe limits for this commonly prescribed medication. There are many prescription analgesics on the market that contain acetaminophen as just one of its ingredients (e.g., Vicodin, Percocet). Physicians may fail to recognize that various prn medications prescribed (often on standing orders) could cumulatively result in toxic amount of acetaminophen. It is not uncommon for physicians to prescribe acetaminophen for fever or mild pain and a combination product with acetaminophen for moderate pain. www.ismp.org/MSAarticles/ref1.htm

1.  Mahlmeister LR. Legal issues and risk management. Best practices in medication administration: Preventing adverse drug events in perinatal settings. *J Perinat Neonat Nurs.* 2007; 21:6-8.
2.  Pastorius D. Crime in the workplace, part 1. *Nurs Manage.* 2007; 38:18-27.
3.  Ulmsten U. Onset and forces of term labor. *Acta Obstetricia et Gynecologica Scandinavica.* 1997; 76:499-514.
4.  Simpson K, Poole J, eds. *Cervical Ripening and Induction and Augmentation of Labor.* Washington, D.C.: Association of Women's Health, Obstetric and Neonatal Nursing; 2002.
5.  Sanchez-Ramos L, Kaunitz AM, Wears RL, Delke L&G,F.L. Misoprostol for cervical ripening and labor induction. *Obstetrics and Gynecology.* 1997; 89:633-642.
6.  American Academy of Pediatrics (AAP) and American College of Obstetricians and Gynecologists (ACOG). *Guidelines for Perinatal Care.* 5th ed. Washington, DC: Author; 2002.
7.  Simpson K, ed. *Cervical Ripening and Induction and Augmentation of Labor.* 2nd ed. Washington, DC: AWHONN; 2002.
8.  American College of Obstetricians and Gynecologists. Induction of labor. Washington, DC: ACOG; 1999; Practice Bulletin No.10:562-569.
9.  Knox GE, Simpson K. High reliability perinatal units: An approach to the prevention of patient injury and medical malpractice claims. *Journal of Healthcare Risk Management.* 1999; 19:24-32.
10. Simpson KR, Knox GE. Common areas of litigation related to care during labor and birth: Recommendations to promote patient safety and decrease risk exposure. *J Perinat Neonat Nurs.* 2003; 17:110-127.
11. Cherouny PH, Federico FA, Haraden C, Leavitt Gullo S, Resar R. Idealized design of perinatal care. IHI innovation series white paper. Cambridge, Massachusetts: Institution for Healthcare Improvement; 2005. Available from: www.IHI.org.
12. Simpson K, Creehan P. *Perinatal Nursing.* 3rd ed. Philadelphia: Lippincott Williams & Wilkins; 2008.
13. Macones GA, Hankins GD, Spong CY, Hauth J, Moore T. The 2008 national institute of child health and human development workshop report on electronic fetal monitoring: Update on definitions, interpretation, and research guidelines. *Obstet Gynecol.* 2008; 112:661-666.
14. Arias F. Pharmacology of oxytocin and prostaglandins. *Clin Obstet Gynecol.* 2000; 43:455-468.
15. Clayworth S. The nurse's role during oxytocin administration. *MCN Am J Matern Child Nurs.* 2000; 25:80-84.
16. Westgate JA, Wibbens B, Bennet L, Wassink G, Parer JT, Gunn AJ. The

intrapartum deceleration in center stage: A physiologic approach to the interpretation of fetal heart rate changes in labor. *Am J Obstet Gynecol.* 2007; 197:236.e1-236.11.

17. Complications follow questionable induction of labor. CRICO/RMF; Available from: http://www.rmf.harvard.edu/high-risk-areas/obstetrics/case-studies/complications. Accessed 12/4/07.

18. ISMP medication safety alert! *Institute for Safe Medication Practices.* Philadelphia: Institute for Safe Medication Practices; 2005;10. Available from: http://www.ismp.org.

19. Simpson KR, Knox GE. Obstetrical accidents involving intravenous magnesium sulfate: Recommendations to promote patient safety. *MCN: The American Journal of Maternal/Child Nursing.* 2004; 29:161-71. (20 ref).

20. Simpson KR. Perinatal patient safety. Minimizing risk of magnesium sulfate overdose in obstetrics. *MCN.* 2006; 31:340.

21. Lehmann CU, Kim GR. Prevention of medication errors. *Clinics in Perinatology.* 2005; 32:107-123.

22. Helm A. *Nursing Malpractice: Sidestepping Legal Minefields.* Philadelphia: Lippincott, Williams & Wilkins; 2003.

23. To err is human: Building a safer health system. Washington DC: National Academy of Science; 1999.

24. Rostant D, Cady R. *Liability Issues in Perinatal Nursing.* Philadelphia: Lippincott; 1999.

25. Smetzer J. Safer medication management. *Nursing Management.* 2001; 32:44-48.

# CHAPTER 7

# Maintaining Competency - Protecting Your Patient and Yourself

*The nurse owes the same duties to self as to others, including the responsibility to preserve integrity and safety, to maintain competence, and to continue personal and professional growth.*

*ANA Code of Ethics for Nurses*

Nursing is a dynamic profession that has undergone many changes over the past years in response to technological advances in health care, consumer demands, and changes in the health care delivery system. Nowhere are these changes more evident than they are in the field of perinatal nursing.[1] In order for safe care to be delivered to both mothers and babies, we need to remain cognizant of the need to have all staff members encouraged in their professional growth, oriented to the policies and procedures of the facility, medication administration, the technology used, emergency procedures and chain of command. Skills need to be continually assessed and in-service education ongoing and supported. Electronic fetal monitoring, documentation and medication administration have been addressed in their respective chapters. The following are further suggestions to maintain competency in caring for mothers and newborns.

**Know Your Institution's Policies and Procedures**

A critical factor in empowering nurses to practice independently within their legislated scope of practice is providing the organizational context that visibly supports that practice. Empowering nurses with decision-making authority must be supported with formalized organizational policies and procedures.[2] Teamwork can be enhanced when every team member knows what is expected. Standardization of key clinical procedures known to increase risk of adverse maternal or fetal outcome is one way to set forth team member expectations.[3]

It makes the patient's attorney's job very easy to prove negligence to a jury when he can present a specific facility policy or procedure as evidence and point out precisely where the care given deviated from it.[4 P-133] This is one reason why it is so important to know your hospital's policies and to be proactive in seeing that they are up-to-date, relevant and clear. Specialty guidelines as published by the Association of Women's Health, Obstetric and Neonatal Nurses (AWHONN), the American Academy of Pediatrics (AAP) and the American College of Obstetricians and Gynecologists (ACOG) should be used.

Policies and procedures should be nurse-friendly (in other words, easily accessible), relevant and not so voluminous that you need vacation time to read them. Helm[4] describes the following characteristics of a good nursing department manual:

➢ General policies and how they apply to the nursing department are explained.

➢ The roles and responsibilities of the nursing department (both internal and in relation to other departments) are outlined.

➢ Handling of emergency situations is addressed.

➢ Consistent terminology is used. When policies and procedures conflict because of inconsistent terms, errors occur, caregivers grow confused, and attorneys can build a case against you and the facility.[5]

It is also important that policies not be absolute. Terms such as *responsible for, shall, and must* impose strict or automatic liability; they do not take into account specific circumstantial factors.[5]

---

**Example of Creating Strict Liability Due to Wording[5]**

A patient may require frequent monitoring of vital signs. The statement, "RNs shall take vital signs every 2 hours," creates strict liability in two areas. First, the RN must handle the vital signs, which may not be necessary. Perhaps an LPN is qualified to take the signs, depending on the patient's condition. This policy does not allow the RN to delegate. Second, the mandate of taking vital signs every 2 hours requires an absolute. What if the RN is not available immediately at precisely the 120-minute mark when the vital signs must be repeated?

A better statement would be: RN or designee will monitor vital signs every 2 hours or as the patient's condition warrants. This allows for delegation and some discretion regarding the frequency of taking vital signs based on the patient's condition.

---

Be proactive in encouraging your facility to create a perinatal practice committee if one does not exist. A perinatal practice committee has two purposes: to establish the basis for and define current institutional practices and to redefine practices accordingly as knowledge, professional guidelines, or regulatory requirements change.[6]

> **Take Home Message**
>
> It is nearly impossible to incorporate a policy and procedure that addresses every potential treatment situation in your facility. But when you deviate from established guidelines, your own words can come back to hurt you.[5]

## Know What is Expected of You as the Charge Nurse

Unfortunately, it is all too frequently that nurses find themselves in charge of a unit without any preparation or orientation to this very important role. Effective charge nurse functioning is essential to safe patient care and the coordination of all team members. The charge nurse must be constantly vigilant of patient census and acuity as well as nurse-to-patient ratios and the skill level of his/her staff.

One of the most crucial duties of the charge nurse is to serve as the first link in the chain of command when unresolved disputes or concerns about patient safety or patient well-being arise. The perinatal charge nurse often makes minute-to-minute, life and death decisions, and timely activation of the chain of command is one of the most important decisions made.[7] The nurse must be prepared to assume such a commanding task and communicate her concerns to nursing management if she does not feel prepared to assume this role. It is imperative that education and support be provided to those assuming the charge role as well as a collaboration with the institution's leadership to develop criteria, an effective orientation and mentoring process, an evaluation tool, and rewards and recognition for charge nurses.[7]

The charge nurse must also have a firm understanding of what tasks may be delegated to other staff members. The specific roles of the registered nurse must be clearly understood and differentiated from the roles of other licensed and unlicensed personnel. Those fundamental responsibilities of assessment, planning, and evaluating patient care that define professional nursing must continue to rest with the registered nurse.[1] Clearly defined parameters for training and supervising unlicensed personnel must be in place. In making the decision to delegate, the likely effects of the activity to be delegated should be assessed, using the following factors:

- potential for harm
- complexity of task
- problem solving and critical thinking required
- unpredictability of outcome
- level of care giver-patient interaction

(For a more comprehensive description, see AWHONN's Clinical Position Statement on The Role of Unlicensed Assistive Personnel in the Care for Women and Newborns in the Additional Resources section.)

---

**Take Home Messages**

If your role expands, your skills have to grow too. If that requires advanced courses, and supervised clinical experience; make sure you get both.

Request a clear, written definition of your role in the hospital. Your hospital should have an overall policy and an individual, written job description for you that specifies the limits of your nursing role. You will be better protected if guidelines for advanced nursing competencies are formally established.

Source: Helm, A. (2003). Nursing Malpractice: Sidestepping Legal Minefields. Lippincott: Philadelphia.

---

## Fulfill all Mandatory Competencies

You have an obligation to fulfill all mandatory competencies as required by your institution. Records of your attendance and completion of these competencies can be obtained by the plaintiff's counsel. Not fulfilling this obligation can prove very problematic should you be named in a lawsuit.

## Medical Record Audits - A Valuable Tool

Auditing medical records is a valuable tool for validating competence. An audit of the medical record provides data about the adherence of the practitioner to hospital policies and procedures, knowledge and compliance with required documentation and can highlight those areas that need further education. It can help to evaluate if care was appropriate based on the patient's chief complaint and also whether critical thinking was used as evidenced by the documented interventions and patient outcomes. The following is a small sample of additional components of a medical record audit:[8]

- Is fetal well-being noted on admission?
- Are appropriate interventions documented during nonreassuring FHR patterns?
- Does the EFM baseline match the documented FHR baseline?
- Are maternal assessments documented during the immediate postpartum period every 15 minutes for the first hour?
- Are newborn assessments documented during the transition to extrauterine life at least every 30 minutes until the newborn's condition has been stable for 2 hours?

## Attain Specialty Certification

Certification gives the obstetric, gynecologic, or neonatal nurse an additional credential that attests to his or her attainment of special knowledge in a specific area beyond the basic nursing degree.[9] Certification measures the command of specialty knowledge and the application of this knowledge as well as demonstrating to colleagues, patients, employers, others in the healthcare field and the public that you are knowledgeable of, experienced in, and committed to nursing practice.[10] Carey's[11] report on the International Study of the Certified Nurse Workforce, suggests that there is evidence that certification may give nurses the means or opportunity to practice in a manner likely to improve patient outcomes, may afford nurses professional growth and financial rewards, such as recognition, reimbursement, salary increase, and career advancement opportunities as well as the opportunity for professional growth. Certified nurses also felt that certification enabled them to experience fewer adverse events and errors in patient care as compared to pre certification. One possible explanation for this is that nurses who seek certification are more motivated to achieve high levels of performance and professionalism.[8]

Attaining certification is not an easy process and involves an initial commitment to review and study the literature pertinent to your specialty area of practice in preparation for undergoing an extensive examination. Some may find this difficult, especially considering the busy lives we lead, but putting the time and energy into properly preparing for the exam will pay off in the end. The examination is usually taken via computer, but some written exams are still possible. After attaining certification, the nurse must also have an ongoing commitment to stay knowledgeable and abreast of current developments because there are educational and practice requirements for certification maintenance. **Table 7-1** is a list of available certifying organizations.

---

**Table 7-1  Organizations That Offer Certification for Perinatal Nurses**

Academy of Certified Birth Educators and Labor Support Professionals (ACBE)
http://www.acbe.com

American Association of Critical Care Nurses (AACN)
http://www.aacn.org

American College of Nurse Midwives (ACNM)
http://www.acnm.org

American Nurses Credentialing Center (ANCC)
http://www.ana.org

International Board of Lactation Consultant Examiners (IBLCE)
http://www.nursingcenter.com

International Childbirth Education Association (ICEA)
http://www.icea.org

Lamaze Childbirth Educator Certification (LCEC)
http://www.lamaze-childbirth.com

National Certification Corporation for the Obstetric, Gynecologic and Neonatal Specialties (NCC)
http://www.nccnet.org

---

**Consider Pursuing Higher Education**

It is never too late to return to school to complete a higher degree of education ( I was 48 years old and computer illiterate when I returned for my Masters). It can be very challenging during those years of raising a family or taking care of aging parents, but it can be done. Even if you chip away at it, one course at a time, you will eventually get there. The rewards and benefits of achieving more education are many and far outweigh the negatives you may face along the way. Along with the self satisfaction that you have reached your goal, your professional life will mature and broaden and more opportunities for professional advancement will present themselves.

## Be Proactive in Initiating and Participating in Practice Drills

Having a baby is a normal physiological function and most of the time everything goes smoothly and without a problem. However, we need to be ready for when things do not go as planned and an emergency arises. Performing drills can be a great way in which to practice the unexpected. Ideally they should be interdisciplinary and as close to reality as possible. The use of simulation has become quite popular and has proven to be a great asset in the learning experience. However, setting up a simulation center can be expensive and not feasible for many institutions. No matter what your resources, the following are some of the emergency situations which should be practiced on a regular basis:

➢ Shoulder dystocia
➢ Maternal/newborn codes
➢ Postpartum hemorrhage
➢ Prolapsed cord
➢ Infant abduction
➢ Stat cesarean birth
➢ Maternal/neonatal seizures

## Membership in Professional Organizations

Join your professional organization. The benefits of being a member of a professional organization are many and include: providing current knowledge of standards and guidelines, networking with colleagues who have the same interest as you in providing safe and competent care to mothers and newborns, high quality conferences and seminars and an opportunity to grow both intellectually and professionally.

There are many opportunities for you to get involved on the local, state and national level within the organization you choose. I recommend starting at the local level and becoming more acquainted with the organization. Volunteering your time and expertise is both beneficial to you and the organization. If you are not comfortable speaking in front of large groups, you can always help behind the scenes with mailing event brochures, helping with registrations and offering your ideas for activities. Advanced degrees are not a requirement - your personal commitment and experience are invaluable and will be greatly appreciated by other members.

## Read, Read, Read

Read to stay current and updated on the changes in practice. I highly recommend the books and articles which I have referenced at the end of each chapter. Simpson, Mahlmeister and Miller address many of the legal issues in our practice today and their articles are often found in the Journal of Obstetrical,

Gynecologic and Neonatal Nursing (JOGNN), the Journal of Perinatal and Neonatal Nursing, The Journal of Maternal/Child Nursing (MCN) and Nursing for Women's Health (formerly AWHONN's Lifelines).

### Guard Against Burnout

Take care of yourself, mentally, physically and spiritually. I know, it is very easy for me to sit and type these words onto paper, but it is so important. Nurses, by nature, are caregivers and nurturers who often look after the needs of everyone else but themselves. After taking care of our families all day long, what do we do? We come into the hospital and work another 8, 10 or 12 hours, often functioning on very little sleep. We work holidays, weekends and rotating shifts. We strive to put on the Martha Stewart Christmas, Thanksgiving and Easter Egg Hunt and admonish ourselves when all does not go as planned. We stress ourselves to be all things to all people. Unfortunately, this constant merry-go-round ride often leads to burnout, depression, resentment and anger which in the end helps no one. It not only affects ourselves, our families and friends, but can also affect our patient care.

As nurses we need to take time and think about what is happening around us. If the position you are in is causing stress due to a poor work environment because of inadequate staffing, doctor/nurse conflict or a non supportive management, *move on*. Take the time to look for another position that will better fit your needs. You may have to travel a little further, but to be able to leave your patients feeling that you have been able to give the care you wanted to and not spend the entire shift in an unpleasant or hostile environment, is well worth it. We need to take time to rejuvenate. We, as healthcare providers, are always on a Give, Give, Give mission and sometimes we just need to give to ourselves so that we can become reenergized so that we can get back to what it is we want to do - take excellent care of our mothers and babies.

1. Rostant D, Cady R. *Liability Issues in Perinatal Nursing.* Philadelphia: Lippincott; 1999.

2. Arford PH. Nurse-physician communication: An organizational accountability. *Nurs Econ.* 2005; 23:72-77.

3. Simpson KR. Failure to rescue: Implications for evaluating quality of care during labor and birth. *J Perinat Neonat Nurs.* 2005; 19:24-36.

4. Helm A. *Nursing Malpractice: Sidestepping Legal Minefields.* Philadelphia: Lippincott, Williams & Wilkins; 2003.

5. Austin S. Legal checkpoints. Policies and procedures: Friend or foe? part 1. *Nurs Manage.* 2001; 32:15.

6. Simpson KR. Strategies for promoting perinatal patient safety: New ideas and methods to measure success. *JOGNN.* 2006; 35:408.

7. Mahlmeister LR. Legal issues and risk management. Best practices in perinatal nursing: Professional role development for charge nurses. *J Perinat Neonat Nurs.* 2006; 20:122-124.

8. Simpson K, Creehan P. *Perinatal Nursing.* 3rd ed. Philadelphia: Lippincott Williams & Wilkins:; 2008.

9. National Certification Corporation for the Obstetric, Gynecologic, and Neonatal Specialities (NCC). *Certification Program.* Chicago: National Council of State Boards of Nursing; 2000.

10. Roman M. Are you certified in your specialty? *Medsurg Nurs.* 2007; 16:219, 237.

11. Cary AH. Certified registered nurses: Results of the study of the certified workforce. *Am J Nurs.* 2001; 101:44-52.

# CHAPTER 8

# When a Lawsuit is Filed

*I found it difficult to see my name in print when I received the legal document (a complaint), several years after caring for this mother and baby. I reacted to it as an attack on my professional judgment and felt offended. I also found it difficult to remember the many complicated aspects of this particular birth, and even more difficult to realize that I was being held accountable for injuries allegedly received.*

M. Patricia Sorich, RNC, BSN[1]

Educational and licensing requirements for nurses increased after World War 11 as nursing tasks became more complex, leading to specialization. These changes meant that nurses began to make independent judgments. Although this increased responsibility provides a more rewarding working environment, it also makes nurses more liable for errors and increases their likelihood of being sued.[2 P-4] Cases involving obstetric errors have at least two plaintiffs: mother and infant. Because the courts recognize a legal duty to the unborn, an obstetric nurse may also be charged with violating the rights of the fetus. Monetary damages tend to be large because of the permanent or long term injuries that can occur to newborns.[2 P-7]

---

**Did You Know?**

The median award in the United States for "medical negligence in child birth cases" is $2.3 million. In 2002, the total U.S. Tort System cost $233 billion and as a result, obstetricians pay some of the highest premiums for malpractice insurance - up to $299,420 per year in some states. Faced with skyrocketing insurance premiums, approximately 1 out of 11 obstetricians nationwide have stopped delivering infants.[3]

From 1998-2007, CRICO/RMF (the patient safety and medical malpractice insurance company owned by and serving the Harvard medical community since 1976) closed 339 malpractice cases involving nurses and paid plaintiffs more than $71 million. CRICO cases opened from 1998-2007 named 373 individual nurses as defendants and represent $173 million in potential losses. While physicians bear the brunt of malpractice allegations, the days of patients being reluctant to sue nurses are gone. (http://www.rmf.harvard.edu)

---

## When a Lawsuit is Filed

**Malpractice Law**

    Malpractice law is part of tort, or personal injury, law. There are three social goals of malpractice litigation: to deter unsafe practices, to compensate persons injured through negligence, and to exact corrective justice. There is a deep-seated tension between the malpractice system and the goals and initiatives of the patient-safety movement.[4] At its root, the problem is one of conflicting cultures: trial attorneys believe that the threat of litigation makes doctors/nurses practice more safely, but the punitive, individualistic, adversarial approach of tort law is antithetical to the non-punitive, systems oriented, cooperative strategies promoted by leaders of the patient-safety movement.[5] To prevail in a tort lawsuit, the plaintiff must prove:

1. The defendant owed a duty of care to the plaintiff. Duty is usually initiated when the nurse is assigned to the patient or, it can be, that the nurse is covering or helping the assigned nurse.
2. There was a breach in this duty and this can be either by omission (i.e. not giving a prescribed medication, not notifying the provider when the fetal heart tracing becomes nonreassuring or not checking the baby bands with the mother to assure that she has the right baby) or commission (i.e. giving the wrong medication or wrong dose, increasing pitocin during hyperstimulation or having the mother breast feed a baby other than her own)
3. Injuries occurred
4. The breach of duty caused the injury/injuries. Determining causation is particularly important in obstetrical malpractice, where it is critical to the outcome of the suit but impossible to determine with certainty.[6]

    The standard traditionally used to evaluate whether the breach in question rises to the level of negligence is the quality of care that would be expected of a reasonably prudent nurse in a similar situation. The standards are the minimal requirements that define an acceptable or satisfactory level of care. The standards of care applied in a professional liability case are typically derived from sources such as state statutes, nurse practice acts, professional associations, professional literature, and the interaction of nursing leaders. In theory there should be no difference in the level of care provided a patient in a teaching hospital compared to the care in a community hospital, or rural hospital compared to a suburban one.[2, 7]

    If a certain practice becomes generally accepted, it will be recognized as a "standard practice." Examples of this include the nurse repeating assessment of an abnormal vital sign and the notification of the physician in the event a patient's condition worsens.[2 P-88] or the initiation of intrauterine resuscitative measures in response to a nonreassuring fetal heart rate tracing. In other words, what is the expected practice in the nursing world? Litigators compare the defendant's behavior with standards established at the time of the alleged negligent act, excluding any changes to the standards that have occurred since the incident.[8] Nurses can be found liable with no liability placed upon the physician. A charge of negligence against a nurse can arise from almost any action or failure to act that results in patient injury - most often an unintentional failure to adhere to a standard of clinical practice - and may lead to a lawsuit.[9] Feutz-Harter[10] cites the case of Brennan v. Orlando Regional Healthcare Systems, Inc., as an example.

---

**Brennan v. Orlando Regional Healthcare Systems, Inc.**
**Case No. 95-2408 (Florida June1999)**

The patient was hospitalized for possible preterm labor. Medications were administered intravenously to attempt to stop the labor. On the 11th day of hospitalization, the IV site (which was the original) was noted to be red, swollen, and a red streak extended 1.5 inches up the patient's arm. The site was changed for the first time. The treating physician was not notified at the time. Three days later, the patient spiked a temperature, went into labor and delivered her baby.

At trial, on behalf of the plaintiffs, the treating physician testified that had he known about the IV site, he would have started the mother on IV antibiotics which would have prevented the staph infection and likely prevented preterm labor and delivery. The plaintiff's nursing expert testified that it was a deviation of the standards of nursing care for the nurses to have left the same IV in place for 11 days and for not notifying the patient's physician and reporting the signs and symptoms of infection. The jury awarded the parents and their 6 year old daughter, $79,728 in past medical expenses, $6,061,996 in future rehabilitation care, $1,505,565 for future loss of wages, and $1,000,000 for future pain and suffering.

---

## Nurses as Defendants in Lawsuits

There are three ways that a practicing nurse can become involved in a lawsuit: as a witness, as an expert, or as a defendant. None of these roles is easy or comfortable for most nurses, but being a defendant is by far the most difficult, threatening and complex.[6]

According to the National Practitioner Data Bank (NPDP), more nurses are being named as defendants in malpractice lawsuits than in the past. The trend shows no signs of stopping, despite efforts by nursing educators to inform nurses and student nurses of their legal and professional responsibilities and limitations. **Tables 8-1 & 8-2** show the liability cases of the Controlled Risk Insurance Company (CRICO) between 1998 and 2007 which involved nurses.

**Table 8-1  CRICO Professional Liability Cases**[11]

| Cases Closed 1998-2007 | All CRICO Cases | All cases involving only nurses | Cases in which physician and a nurse were named |
|---|---|---|---|
| Total Cases | 2,338 | 339 | 150 |
| Cases closed with indemnity payment | 31% | 47% | 53% |
| Total indemnity payment | $375 M | $71 M | $56 M |
| Average indemnity payment | $521,000 | $441,000 | $709,000 |
| Cases closed with indemnity payment >$ 1M | 125 (5%) | 21 (6%) | 17 (11%) |

**Table 8-2  CRICO Cases Involving Nurses**[11]
1998-2007 (N-364 cases)/Total Defendants - N=1,132

| Institution/Organization | 321 |
|---|---|
| Physician | 387 |
| Nurse | 373 |
| ❖  Registered Nurse | ❖  297 |
| ❖  Nurse Practitioner | ❖  41 |
| ❖  Certified Nurse Midwife | ❖  29 |
| ❖  Licensed Practical Nurse | ❖  3 |
| ❖  Nurse Assistant | ❖  2 |
| ❖  CRNA | ❖  1 |

While individual practitioners have a duty to the patient, the hospital also has duties which include:[2 P-37]

1. A duty to use reasonable care in the maintenance of safe and adequate facilities and equipment
2. A duty to select and retain competent physicians
3. A duty to oversee all persons who practice medicine within the purview as to patient care
4. A duty to formulate, adopt, and enforce adequate rules and policies to ensure quality care for patients

**The Litigation Process**

Today's technology has lulled many couples into a false sense that they can only deliver the perfect child - with the athletic ability of Tiger Woods, the brilliance of Bill Gates or the drop dead good looks of Jennifer Lopez. However, despite ever-improving knowledge, technology and technique in labor and delivery, there will always be babies born with complications. Families of a compromised newborn encounter many reactions and emotions, including surprise, sadness, disappointment, anger, grief and guilt. Given the nature of these reactions and emotions, the family's first reaction is not that of filing a lawsuit. It is when their hurt turns into confusion and distrust that they seek the advice of an attorney.[12]

Other factors that may influence a patient to file a claim of malpractice include: a poor relationship with the healthcare provider or clinician; television advertising by law firms; explicit recommendations by health providers or professionals to seek legal advice; the impression of not being kept informed by the healthcare provider or clinician and financial concerns.[13]

The litigation process can be very complex and run over the course of many years. (**Figure 8-1**). The following are steps that the trial process usually follows:[7]

➤ The parents seek the advice and services of an attorney.
➤ The attorney reviews the information he has obtained from the parents and requests the medical records.
➤ A *complaint* is filed. A *complaint* is a written formal statement of the plaintiff's claim.
➤ The lawsuit is initiated when the complaint is filed with the court.
➤ The defendant receives a copy of the complaint and summons, either by certified mail or by a process server. **At this time, the nurse should immediately notify his/her supervisor, hospital risk management and insurance carrier. DO NOT CONTACT THE PLAINTIFF OR HER ATTORNEY.**
➤ *Discovery* begins. *Discovery* is a process used to obtain relevant information about the case prior to trial. It allows both sides to evaluate the opposition's strengths and weaknesses and whether a trial is in their best interest. Methods for discovery include:
1. Oral deposition
2. Written deposition
3. Interrogatories - written questions sent from one party to another that must be answered under oath. Unlike depositions, interrogatories can only be obtained from a party to the action and the answers prepared in writing. Interrogatories must be answered within a time period established by state law. The questions are answered by the party and

When a Lawsuit is Filed

Figure 8-1     Lawsuit Pathway

The Suit is Filed

Investigation of Medical Records, Evaluation of Damages, Liability & Negligence

Discovery - Interrogatories, Depositions

The Suit May be Either Settled with Payment or Dropped at This Time

Alternative Dispute Resolution (Binding Arbitration) is another method which could end in settlement

TRIAL

The Players: Judge, Plaintiff & Attorney, Defendant & Attorney, Expert Witnesses, Fact Witnesses

VERDICT

Settled with Payment

Suit dismissed

Reference: Association of Women's Health, Obstetric and Neonatal Nurses (1999). Liability issues in perinatal nursing. Philadelphia: Lippincott.

reviewed by the attorney before the party signs under oath.

4. Requests for production and inspection of documents and other items
5. Physical and mental examinations

➤ Potential experts for the physicians, the hospital, and the nurses are contacted to begin reviewing records.

➤ Experts are named and depositions taken

➤ If no settlement is reached after negotiations between plaintiff and defendant attorneys, a court date is set. A case can settle at any time prior to or during the trial. **Remember that settlement is not an admission of guilt or negligence, but a formal agreement to end the legal dispute.**

### Statutes of Limitations

Statutes of limitations establish time limits within which a patient or someone acting on behalf of the patient must file a claim in response to an injury. These time limits are defined by state law and vary from state to state. Sometimes it is not possible to identify the cause of an injury or to discover that an injury has occurred. Depending on the circumstances, the time period may begin when the injury occurred, when it was first discovered, or at the end of treatment.[14] Childbirth injuries are usually accorded a much longer time period than other injuries due to the child's ongoing growth and development and the need to assess delays and/or accomplishments.

### The Deposition

The deposition is an examination of a witness under oath with each attorney asking questions in the presence of a court reporter who records the questions and answers.[7 P-54] As part of the discovery process, depositions are also an opportunity for attorneys on both sides to evaluate the credibility of you, potential witnesses and others who may testify in court.[15] The deposition may take place in a variety of locations (i.e. hospital conference room, attorney's office, hotel conference room). Although depositions are not conducted in the formality of a courtroom nor is a judge present, they are extremely important. The testimony rendered at a deposition may determine whether an action will be perused, settled, or dismissed.[10]

Being deposed is not a pleasant experience. Believe me when I say, a root canal has more appeal. However, you can and will get through it. Important things you want to remember about the deposition:

1. They can be long and tedious. Try to get a good nights rest before.
2. Expect to be nervous - you would not be normal if you did not feel some anxiety. Attorneys can be very intimidating, but they should not be allowed to abuse you. Try to use relaxation techniques that work for you.

3. Always have an attorney with you.

4. Dress professionally.

5. Be honest and truthful - do not even think about concealing information or lying. One answer shown to be untruthful can discredit all of your testimony and you can be charged with perjury. If you do find that you have made a mistake, correct it *immediately. Do not leave the deposition without correcting any mistakes that you have come to realize, no matter when they occurred during the deposition.*

6. Avoid adjectives or superlatives such as "I never" or "I always" as they may come back to haunt you.

7. Never let the opposing attorney put words into your mouth.

8. Do not make any attempts at jokes or levity.

9. "Off the record" does not exist. If you have any conversation with anybody in the deposition room, be prepared for questions on that conversation.

10. Remember that the attorney deposing you is just doing their job and try not to take questions too personally.

11. **BE PREPARED**. Review the medical records before hand and ask your attorney what to expect.

12. **Practice** describing your standards. You need to confidently show that you know the standards. Be sure to *emphasize* that any adaptation to the standard was done because of individual patient need.

13. Exercise your patient advocacy skills on behalf of yourself - insisting on information, requesting periodic updates from counsel or administration, and asking to be put in contact with people who can supply information, perspective, and support.[6]

14. Understand the question. Listen and pay attention to what it is you are being asked. If you do not understand the question, you must ask the questioner to make the question crystal clear before you answer it. Many problems arise from failure to understand the question.

15. If you do not know an answer to a question, say you do not, DO NOT GUESS. "I do not recall" is perfectly acceptable. Beware of answering "no" as that means absolutely not. "I do not recall" means exactly that and may be more accurate.

16. Answer only the questions asked - DO NOT OFFER INFORMATION. You do not know where the attorney will take it. Believe me when I say, they are very, very clever and I do not mean that in a devious way, but they know how to elicit information and can take you down a path you really did not want to be on.

17. Ask for a break if you need one. After hours of questioning, you can start to feel totally exhausted.

18. Questions may seem repetitive and make no sense to you, but you need to answer them to the best of your ability. Maintain your composure and do not become angry or defensive.

19. Remember that most questions are fair game unless your attorney objects (however, they can still object and then tell you to answer - I still have not figured that one out) Questions, besides your name, address, date of birth and education, most likely will include:

   ➤ Describing the orientation you received to the unit on which the situation occurred.

   ➤ Any classes you may have attended.

   ➤ Name of the instructor who taught the classes.

   ➤ Your knowledge of your hospital's policies - do they exist, where are they located and when is the last time you accessed them.

   ➤ The specific care you rendered to the patient.

   ➤ What or if you belong to any professional organizations.

   ➤ What professional journals you subscribe to if any.

   ➤ If the case involves electronic fetal monitoring, be prepared to spend a great amount of time describing the strip. You may be asked to describe the fetal heart rate baseline, decelerations, the variability, any reassuring or nonreassuring signs and your reasoning behind any actions taken or not taken.

   ➤ Be prepared for questions regarding pathophysiology that may apply to the case. For example: What is preeclampsia? What are the signs and symptoms of worsening preeclampsia? How does the mother's condition affect the fetus?

   ➤ Be prepared to answer questions regarding any medications your patient received.

   ➤ Your documentation will be dissected. Be prepared to describe intrauterine resuscitative measures and why you did or did not document them.

   ➤ Be prepared to talk about your Chain of Command policy.

**Will A Personal Journal Help You in Court or During a Deposition?**

Some nurses record workplace events in a personal journal in case they are sued. Lawyers disagree as to whether this practice is helpful or harmful. Remember that the opposing attorney may use it to discredit you should it conflict with the medical record. If you do decide to keep a journal, follow these guidelines:[16]

- ➤ Keep it factual.
- ➤ Keep it objective. Documenting defamatory or nasty comments could embarrass you if your journal is subpoenaed by the court.
- ➤ Keep it safe.
- ➤ Be truthful about its existence. Your attorney will review it to see if it could cause you problems in court.

---

**Examples of Potentially Harmful Responses Taken from Nurse Depositions**

#1

Attorney: Am I correct, Nurse Johnson, in saying that Mrs. A. was admitted to the hospital for an induction of labor and you were assigned to her care?

Nurse: Yes.

Attorney: Nurse Johnson, according to the record, Mrs. A. received Cytotec. Please tell me what cytotec is used for.

Nurse: I haven't a clue since I do not put it into the patient. The doctor does.

#2

Attorney: Nurse Smith, do you belong to any professional organizations.

Nurse: No.

Attorney: Nurse Smith, do you regularly subscribe to or read any professional journals?

Nurse: No.

Attorney: Nurse Smith, do you refer to any particular textbooks on maternity nursing and if so which ones?

Nurse: No. I did have a textbook once, but I have not seen it for a long time.

Attorney: Nurse Smith, does the hospital make any textbooks available to you?

Nurse: Maybe, but I really do not know.

Attorney: Nurse Smith, do you attend any seminars or conferences related to your work in labor and delivery?

Nurse: Not if I have to pay for them.

---

#3

| | |
|---|---|
| Attorney: | Nurse White, did you consider questioning Dr. Jones as to his orders to increase the pitocin in view of the fact that you just told me, when we were looking at the fetal monitoring tracing, that your patient was having contractions every minute and the fetal heart rate was 180 with minimal variability? |
| Nurse: | No, I do not question doctor's orders. They are in charge of the patient and it is my job to follow orders. |

#4

| | |
|---|---|
| Attorney: | Nurse Brown, and certainly, at least I guess, at 6 o'clock the presence of continued decelerations was concerning to you since you noted the M.D. was aware of it? |
| Nurse: | Right. At this point I wanted - I wanted to point out, if, you know, in my chart that the M.D. was aware of the pattern. |
| Attorney: | There was nothing - there is an absence of any response, at least in your chart after you say that the M.D. is aware of the pattern. Do we take that to mean that there were instructions given to you by Dr. T. in response to the presence of continued variable decelerations? |
| Nurse: | It is hard to say just based on what I'm looking at. |
| Attorney: | Well, I mean, is there anything anywhere in the chart at 6 a.m. when you made sure that Dr. T. was aware of the situation that she gave you any order, told you anything to address that? |
| Nurse: | It doesn't say anywhere according to, just looking at the chart, what was said at 6 a.m. |

## The Trial

It is typical to have many delays and postponements as a case moves toward trial. This increases the stress to defendants and makes it difficult to prepare for trial. Physical and emotional manifestations of stress are common and are exacerbated by the length of time that defendants are involved in the process without progress or resolution.[6]

In the event that a case goes forward to trial, you must be prepared for being questioned by both the plaintiff and defense attorneys. Recognize that the role of the opposing attorney is to discredit, confuse, point out ambiguities and differences in opinion, and to destroy confidence. This is not a personal attack but is for the benefit of the jury and the attorney's client.[10] Many of the points I have listed regarding preparing and weathering a deposition apply to testifying in court, but now you will be in front of a jury and your demeanor, preparation and ability to explain your role in the case must be able to convince the jury to render a verdict in your favor.

Remember that jurors have a great amount of respect for nurses and feel that a trusting relationship exists between a nurse and her patient. That trusting relationship also invokes a willingness to forgive mistakes or accept unfortunate results. However, if the jurors perceive that the trust has been violated, they will react with a strong empathic sense of betrayal that results in moral outrage and indignation. You must work to maintain that trust.[10]

## The Expert Witness

In the majority of medical malpractice actions brought against nurses, it is required that a nurse expert witness render testimony to establish the appropriate standard of care and to identify how the defendant nurse deviated from that standard.[17 P-338] The expert witness plays an important role in presenting nursing standards for the jury to consider. The expert nurse's duty is to present to the jury what the nursing standards were at the time the incident took place and to give an opinion as to whether the nurse adhered to the standards and acted as a reasonable prudent nurse would have in a similar situation.[7 P-34] A nurse must meet certain criteria to be considered as an expert witness[2, 17 P-212] This includes:

➢ Current licensure to practice nursing
➢ Qualified by education, experience, employment, publications, or research to render an opinion
➢ Credentials must match or exceed the defendant's
➢ Clinical expertise in the same specialty as the defendant
➢ Ability to explain complex information to a lay jury so that they can understand it and make a decision
➢ Ability to remain calm while opposing attorney tries to discredit or minimize your testimony
➢ Lack of bias

## Characteristics of Nurses at Risk for a Lawsuit

Just as certain characteristics of physicians at risk for a lawsuit have been described in the literature, Helm[2] describes the following characteristics of a nurse who is likely to be a defendant in a lawsuit. The nurse:

➢ Lacks sensitivity to the patient's complaints or fails to take them seriously
➢ Fails to identify and meet the patient's emotional and physical needs
➢ Refuses to recognize the limits of her nursing skills and personal competency
➢ Lacks sufficient education for the task and responsibilities associated

with specific practice setting
- ➢ Displays an authoritarian and inflexible attitude when providing care
- ➢ Inappropriately delegates responsibilities to subordinates

In contrast, it is my opinion that the nurse who is *least likely* to find themselves as a defendant in a lawsuit demonstrates a *commitment* to:

- ➢ Evidence based practice
- ➢ Always acting as a patient advocate
- ➢ Respecting the patient's culture, race and religion
- ➢ Being a team player
- ➢ Improving communication among team members
- ➢ Initiating the Chain of Command when her patient's well being is in jeopardy
- ➢ Following the 5 rights of medication administration
- ➢ Delegating tasks appropriately; knowing the limitations and strengths of those to whom tasks are delegated
- ➢ Using equipment properly
- ➢ Following rules of good documentation
- ➢ Following hospital policy, local and national standards
- ➢ Remaining current by being a member of her professional organization
- ➢ Completing all competencies
- ➢ Speaking up when she is given duties for which she lacks the skill or knowledge. Remember that medication errors are among the most common causes of patient harm and subsequent lawsuits stemming from floating.[16] (We need to be proactive when unreasonable demands, such as floating to an unfamiliar specialty, are placed on us. In these days of advanced technology and patient acuity, the belief that "*A nurse is a nurse, is a nurse*" is not only outdated, but a set up for error and significant harm to the patient.)

**Malpractice Insurance - To Have or Have Not - That is the Question**

| Types of Insurance Policies | |
| --- | --- |
| Claims made | This type of policy covers you only while it is in effect. In other words, in order to be covered, the claim has to be made or a lawsuit filed while the policy is active. If the policy lapses, you are not covered. |
| Occurrence | This policy covers you for incidents that occur while the policy is in effect BUT does not have to be active when a claim is made or a lawsuit is filed. If the policy lapses, you are still covered. |

I am often asked if it is wise to carry malpractice insurance and, honestly,

## When a Lawsuit is Filed

I have not come up with a firm decision (although I do carry insurance) because I have read conflicting theories about it. I will take the coward's way out and present both sides of the story and let you decide. There is a misconception that nurses with malpractice insurance get sued more often than nurses without it. In reality, plaintiffs do not know who is insured until after a lawsuit is filed: that information is shared during discovery. Some nurses also fear that the employer may attempt to recover losses should the nurse be found negligent. This is called *indemnification and contribution*. There is limited data to support this, but it has been tried. Two valid reasons why a healthcare institution would not or should not sue nurses are 1) the nurse works under the control of the institution and it is responsible for the nurse's actions and 2) it makes for very poor public relations should an institution sue its own nurses.[18 P-46]

The American Association of Nurse Attorneys strongly recommends that no nurse be without insurance protection. Reasons to carry insurance include:[19]

> - If you are reported to the board of nursing for either malpractice or misconduct, you will need insurance for legal representation because you are on your own. An employer's policy will usually *only* cover you for malpractice representation.
> - Although it is extremely rare, if there is a judgment against you and it is not satisfied, your assets can be seized.
> - Your employer's policy will not cover you or anything happening outside of work or for allegations of departure from the institution's policies and procedures.
> - If you believe that the attorney appointed by your employer's insurance company has a conflict of interest (i.e. if you violate a hospital policy or procedure and the insurance excludes coverage of you due to this behavior) and sense that he will be looking out for the hospital's best interest and not yours, you may need to pay for your own attorney.[15]

Reasons cited for not carrying insurance include:[20]

> - When you are acting within the scope of your job description and your nursing license and are not engaged in criminal activity, your employer bears vicarious liability for any mistake you make.
> - Your hospital purchases professional liability (in the millions of dollars) for itself and its employees. It is in their best interest that you are insured.
> - Attorneys rarely go after a person's assets.
> - Plaintiff notification of an additional source of money may cause a nurse to stay within a lawsuit when they would otherwise have been dropped. (I did see evidence of this in one case in which a travel nurse was retained

in the case after others had been dismissed so that the agency she was employed by could be named. In reviewing the case, she actually had very little contact with the patient and it was clearly a bogus allegation to name her. The case was finally dropped, but not until a very long time had passed and we were preparing to go to trial.)

If you do decide to have professional liability insurance, it is recommended that the nurse investigate what policies are available. Nurses may not even be aware that their institution provides an amount of liability coverage for them as the premiums are not deducted from paychecks. Selection of a policy is an individual decision and guided by a nurse's scope of practice which determines risk and coverage.[7] Rostant[7] further proposes the following guidelines:

- ➢ Discuss institutional coverage provided by your employer with the risk manger; obtain a copy for your records if possible
- ➢ Assess the commercial market through professional organizations, insurance agent, and colleagues
- ➢ Compare premiums
- ➢ Identify your exposure; compare the job description with the scope of practice limits in your state
- ➢ Insure for the biggest exposures and broadest coverage
- ➢ Check the insurance carrier's financial standing
- ➢ Determine if there are any premium reductions for educational attendance
- ➢ Investigate whether the insurance company provides additional services such as consultations, newsletters, educational programs, or any insurance reports
- ➢ The insurance application is a legal document. If you provide any false information, it may void the policy[21]
- ➢ If you are involved in nursing administration, education, research, or advanced or nontraditional nursing practice, be especially careful in selecting a policy because routine policies may not cover these activities[21]

**Nurses Need to Know About the Law and Ethics**

When speaking about how far nursing has come as a profession, I have been known to say to colleagues that it is almost a compliment to be sued (I know, sounds sick and they look at me aghast). But my point being, we are now *finally* being recognized as professionals who are capable of critical thinking and independence. We are no longer the "handmaidens" or "borrowed servants" of the physician, stoking the fires to keep our patients warm, but educated, professional people who are expected to take responsibility for those placed in our care. (In Victorian times, a "good nurse" was considered one who came to work sober and stayed so during her entire shift!) We should be very proud of our accomplishments since it has taken eons to get to this point and protect what we as a profession have worked so hard to achieve.

We have seen many changes in our healthcare delivery system and with this have come great opportunities for nursing. However, these opportunities are accompanied by great responsibilities for legal and ethical decision making and greater exposure to legal liability. Nurses must be educated about the law and ethics to be armed with the tools necessary for professional survival.[22] Becoming an active member of your professional organization, attending national conventions, networking with professionally active colleagues, attending seminars and in-services and reading the legal and/or ethics section of specialty nursing journals are just a few ways in which to accomplish this need.

---

**Take Home Message**

The best defense against malpractice claims is prevention or minimization of harm whenever possible, through adherence to evidence-based practice guidelines. Professional organizations such as ACOG and AWHONN have developed a number of practice guidelines and position statements. The challenge is ensuring that these guidelines are used consistently by a care team that works together smoothly and effectively and complemented by complete and accurate documentation of that care.[23, 24]

---

1. Sorich M, Letizia M. Nursing malpractice litigation: A personal journey. *Maternal Child Nursing.* 1994; 19: 249-254.
2. Helm A. *Nursing Malpractice: Sidestepping Legal Minefields.* Philadelphia: Lippincott, Williams & Wilkins; 2003.
3. Hankins GD, MacLennan AH, Speer ME, Strunk A, Nelson K. Obstetric litigation is asphyxiating our maternity services. *Obstet Gynecol.* 2006; 107:1382-1385.
4. Studdert DM, Mello MM, Brennan TA. Medical malpractice. *NEJM.* 2004; 350: 283-292.
5. Bovbjerg R, Miller R, Shapiro D. Paths to reducing medical injury: Professional liability and discipline vs. patient safety--and the need for a third way. *J Law Med Ethics.* 2001; 29:369-380.
6. Rhodes AM. Malpractice litigation. *MCN.* 1994; 19: 257.
7. Rostant D, Cady R. *Liability Issues in Perinatal Nursing.* Philadelphia: Lippincott; 1999.
8. Showers JL. Protection from negligence lawsuits. *Nurs Manage.* 1999; 30:23-28.
9. Croke EM. Nurses, negligence, and malpractice: An analysis based on more than 250 cases against nurses. *Am J Nurs.* 2003; 103:54-64.
10. Feutz-Harter S. The legal system and principles. In: *Legal and Ethical Standards for Nurses.* Eau Claire, Wisconsin: Professional Education Systems, Inc.; 2006:5-36.
11. Hoffman J, Yu W. Medical malpractice cases involving nurses (and often physicians). *Forum.* 2008; 28:3-5.
12. Holder WL. Shark-proof your practice. how the law is every nurse's best ally. *AWHONN Lifelines.* 1997; 1:53-57.
13. Oyebode F. Clinical errors and medical negligence. *Advances in Psychiatric Treatment.* 2006; 12:221-227.
14. Ferrell KG. Documentation, part 2: The best evidence of care. Complete and accurate charting can be crucial to exonerating nurses in civil lawsuits. *Am J Nurs.* 2007; 107:61-64.
15. Brooke PS. So you've been named in a lawsuit?: What happens next?. *Nursing.* 2006; 36:44-48.
16. Goldberg K, ed. *Surefire Documentation: How, what, and when Nurses Need to Document.* St. Louis: Mosby; 1999.
17. Feutz-Harter S. *Nursing and the Law.* 6th ed. Wisconsin: Professional Education Systems, Inc.; 1997.
18. Simpson K, Creehan P. *Perinatal Nursing.* 2nd ed. Philadelphia: Lippincott; 2001.

19. Brous EA. Malpractice insurance and licensure protection. *Am J Nurs.* 2008; 108:34-36.

20. Craig PA, Miller LA. Should nurses purchase their own professional liability insurance? *MCN Am J Matern Child Nurs.* 1998; 23:123-124.

21. Holmes H, ed. *Nurse's Legal Handbook.* 4th ed. Pennsylvania: Springhouse; 2000.

22. Ely-Pierce K. A call to arms. *JONAS Healthc Law Ethics* Regul. 1999; 1:5-7.

23. Simpson KR, Knox GE. Common areas of litigation related to care during labor and birth: Recommendations to promote patient safety and decrease risk exposure. *J Perinat Neonat Nurs.* 2003; 17:110-127.

24. Cherouny PH, Federico FA, Haraden C, Leavitt Gullo S, Resar R. Idealized design of perinatal care. IHI innovation series white paper. Cambridge, Massachusetts: Institution for Healthcare Improvement; 2005. Available from: www.IHI.org.

# Case Studies

**Case Study**

**Unprepared for Labor and Delivery Worst Case Scenario**

<u>Clinical Sequence</u>

The 25-year-old mother of a three-year-old was scheduled for induction to deliver twin boys at her community hospital. Her pregnancy was uncomplicated, except that the non-presenting twin was in a breech presentation. In planning the delivery, the obstetrician requested portable ultrasound equipment and asked Anesthesia to be on hand.

Following induction via Pitocin, the first twin was delivered vaginally, without difficulty. When the obstetrician encountered problems delivering the second fetus, he re-confirmed that it was still a breech presentation. During an attempt to turn the baby via internal cephalic version, the obstetrician intentionally ruptured the membranes. The umbilical cord was wrapped around the baby's feet and lower body. As the obstetrician further attempted to re-position the baby head-first for a vaginal delivery, the cervix contracted on his hand. The anesthesiologist, who had been called away, was called back to administer nitrous oxide to relax the uterus for further attempts to reposition the baby.

No ultrasound equipment was present in the delivery room, so the nurse monitored the fetal heart rate with a hand held device. At one point, while the obstetrician was attempting to reposition the second twin, the fetal heart rate dropped to 43 BPM. After eight minutes and no successs at turning the fetus, the obstetrician called for a cesarean section.

The baby was born with very low Apgars, no gag reflex, and an EEG demonstrated severe brain damage. He was diagnosed with spastic quadriplegia, was blind and died five months after birth.

<u>Allegation</u>

The parents sued the obstetrician, alleging negligent delays in delivery and treatment of fetal distress.

## Case Studies

Disposition

Expert reviews for the defense were mixed, but the jury returned a verdict for the defense.

Analysis

1. Although the obstetrician prevailed at trial, the defense cited a lack of adequate planning for any untoward events as a problem in this case. Even though he requested Anesthesia and ultrasound just in case he would need them, they were not there when he actually needed them.

   *Planning ahead can be approached either from the perspective that "things usually work out well," or "let's prepare for what might go wrong." If you focus on what is most likely to occur - what a reasonable person would do - you satisfy the letter of the law but miss the opportunity to go one level beyond that and prepare for the worst case scenario. Planning for what - and who - you expect to be in the room when a crisis "could" occur is the first level of vigilance. Systems and teamwork which make certain those things actually are present - with some form of redundancy - provide a second level of safety and peace of mind.*

2. The decision to rupture the membranes, without access to ultrasound monitoring in the delivery room, was questioned by experts who reviewed the case. The obstetrician had requested it, but the nurse was unable to locate the portable machine.

   *When it is unreasonable to supply an often used piece of equipment in every room, the clinicians who use that equipment need to work out a policy or protocol that assure it is available when needed.*

3. The obstetrician in this case proceeded on a course for a second vaginal delivery without seeking or receiving advice from another clinician. In the eyes of the jury, that was not substandard practice, but a team approach might have led to a different decision when the repositioning attempts were unsuccessful.

   *The major attribute of team training is communication between various health care professionals on a level playing field. Communication among colleagues is respected as motivated by a common goal rather than competition or hierarchy. Asking for help and offering advice and assistance, are seen as acts of team strength, not individual faults.*

4. In a medical malpractice lawsuit, the jury is asked to determine if the physician's actions were reasonable for that specialty and time. The jury in this case decided the obstetrician acted reasonably in continuing to attempt a vaginal delivery of the second twin.

*It is hard to judge judgment. Physicians are expected, by the court at least, to behave as other reasonable physicians would: not like the best physician, but not like the worst. But while a jury might fulfill its obligation with a judgment of "reasonable" (i.e. average), medicine owes it to the patient population to strive for better. Only when preventable injuries no longer occur does anyone actually win.*

(http://www.rmf.harvard.edu/case-studies)

Case Studies

**Case Study**

**Failure to Treat Signs and Symptoms of Fetal Distress**

Clinical Sequence

In January 2000, the plaintiffs were expecting the birth of their third child. The prior two pregnancies had been complicated by premature and difficult deliveries. The plaintiff was very concerned about this pregnancy and stated she wanted a cesarean section delivery to avoid any of the problems she had experienced with her prior deliveries. A cerclage was used in order to carry the pregnancy to term but rather than schedule a cesarean section the defendant obstetrician elected to induce the plaintiff using Pitocin. On January 22, 2000, the plaintiff mother was admitted to the hospital for induction of labor with the use of Pitocin. Pitocin was begun at approximately 10:30 a.m. and the plaintiff was under the care of her obstetrician and three labor room nurses (all of whom were defendants). Pitocin was periodically increased and contractions began.

Beginning at 11:32 a.m. and continuing until approximately 1:42 p.m. the defendant nurses were noting frequent contractions with variable decelerations of the fetal heart rate as low as 80 beats per minute. By 1:55 p.m. the nurses noted that the variable decelerations had a late component and the plaintiff had begun leaking green meconium stained amniotic fluid. Between 1:55 p.m. and 3:15 p.m. the nursing documentation notes non-repetitive late decelerations of the fetal heart rate. The defendant obstetrician evaluated the plaintiff on at least three occasions between 12:25 p.m. and 3:15 p.m. and was aware of the worrisome changes in the fetal heart rate and the presence of meconium, yet no steps were taken to stop the Pitocin or get the baby delivered.

Starting at 3:30 p.m. until the time of delivery at 7:18 p.m., the nurses and obstetricians continued to note the presence of late decelerations with slow return to base line as well as minimal long term variability. Despite these findings, delivery was not expedited, the plaintiff was not offered a cesarean section delivery and the Pitocin continued.

The plaintiff delivered her baby at 7:18 p.m. He was significantly depressed at birth with Apgars of 2, 6, and 7. He was not breathing and required assisted ventilation and oxygen. Within 8 hours after birth, the baby began exhibiting seizures, which were treated with Phenobarbital. He was transferred to Children's Hospital on 1/23/00 for further management of his seizures. A head MRI performed on 1/28/00 showed findings consistent with HIE (hypoxic ischemic encephalopathy). Further complications were also attributed to HIE and birth asphyxia. The child cannot walk, talk or sit unsupported. He requires a feeding tube and assistance with all aspects of daily living. He will never live independently.

The plaintiffs were prepared to present expert testimony that there were signs of fetal distress requiring delivery as early as 1:40 p.m. and the defendants failed to respond to these signs with intrauterine resuscitation and cesarean section delivery. As a result, the plaintiff's experts were prepared to testify that the baby suffered a prolonged decrease of oxygen to the brain resulting in his profound brain damage at birth.

The defendants were prepared to present expert testimony that there was not evidence on the fetal monitor strips that warranted earlier delivery via cesarean section and that the baby's presentation at birth did not account for the severe injuries he went on to display and that it was more likely the child suffered some injury before his mother presented to the hospital for induction.

The case settled after mediation for $4,900,000.

(http://www.lubinandmeyer.com/cases/cerebralpalsy)

**Case Study**

**Failure to Diagnose and Treat Signs and Symptoms of Persistent Fetal Distress Resulting in Brain Damage**

In April of 2001, the plaintiff was expecting the birth of her second child on or about 4/14/01. Prenatal testing, including non-stress testing and biophysical profiles, all showed a well-developed, healthy baby. On 4/11/01, the defendant obstetrician admitted the plaintiff to the hospital for cervical ripening and Pitocin induction. The Pitocin was started at 6:00 a.m. on 4/12/01 and at approximately 9:31 a.m., the plaintiff spontaneously ruptured her membranes. The labor continued without complications until approximately 3:20 p.m. when the baby's heart rate began to show persistent late decelerations. At 4:50 p.m., the fetal heart rate pattern became even more non-reassuring with decreased variability. Despite being aware of these worrisome signs, the defendant obstetrician allowed the labor to continue.

Throughout the afternoon and evening, the plaintiff was also cared for by the two defendant nurses. These defendant nurses recognized the problems in the baby's heart rate, gave the plaintiff oxygen, turned her from side to side but continued the Pitocin. The patient pushed for almost three hours. During that time, the plaintiffs were prepared to present evidence at trial that there was clear evidence of fetal distress and the defendants failed to intervene. At 12:03 a.m. on 4/13/01 - almost nine hours after problems were noted - the child was delivered. She needed to be resuscitated in the delivery room and then was sent immediately to the NICU where she needed to be intubated. The child was found to have seizures and a brain CT scan showed the child had suffered a subarachnoid hemorrhage. She currently is severely developmentally delayed and has spastic quadriparesis. She is unable to speak, walk, feed herself and is legally blind.

The case settled at mediation for $5,000,000.

(http://www.lubinandmeyer.com/cases/cerebralpalsy)

**Case Study**

**Results Recorded for a Test Not Performed**

<u>Clinical Sequence</u>

A 30-year-old woman, pregnant with her third child (G3, P1, TAB 1) was followed by a nurse practitioner (NP) throughout her uneventful pregnancy. The same NP had cared for her during her prior pregnancy. The patient was healthy with no risk factors and had no complications with her prior pregnancy and delivery. At eight weeks, she began routine prenatal care at a hospital-based clinic.

At 11 weeks, the NP counseled the patient regarding optional alpha-fetoprotein (AFP) and HIV tests. The patient was informed that the AFP, which may identify spina bifida and Down's syndrome, is usually performed between the 15th and 18th week of the pregnancy. She was further instructed that patients whose AFP is abnormal typically undergo additional testing such as ultrasound and amniocentesis to aid a more definitive diagnosis. (During her pregnancy, this patient's AFP test had been normal.)

At 16 weeks, the patient was seen by a third-year resident. Her examination was normal and the baby's size was appropriate for its age. The physician ordered a growth ultrasound for 18 weeks but did not order the AFP, which typically would have been done at this visit.

At her scheduled visit at 20 weeks, the patient saw the NP who reviewed her record and noted that an ultrasound performed at 18 weeks indicated a normal fetus. The NP also documented that an AFP had been performed at 18 weeks indicated a normal fetus. The patient received routine care for the remainder of her pregnancy. Following delivery, the baby was diagnosed with Down's syndrome and a cardiac anomaly which required cardiac surgery a year later. The clinicians met with the parents and explained that the AFP results (from her first pregnancy) in her record had been errantly interpreted as being the results of a test during her third pregnancy.

The family filed suit against the nurse practitioner and two physicians for wrongful birth based on their failure to do appropriate prenatal testing.

The case was settled in the mid-range ($100,000-$499,000) with the liability assessed equally to the NP and the resident.

# Case Studies

<u>Analysis</u>

1.  The AFP test result from the first pregnancy was inappropriately filed in the medical record leading the NP to assume that this was the test for the current pregnancy.

    *A quality audit of medical records can reduce opportunities for misinterpretation, such as confusing dates. Given the chance for errors, even with electronic medical records, staff training should reinforce the importance of precise reading and review of the chart, particularly when reviewing data that may have a direct impact on the treatment plan and recommendations for the patient.*

2.  At 11 weeks, the NP failed to document in the medical record whether or not the patient intended to have the AFP test at her next visit. The resident's note did not mention the AFP either.

    *Even for optional testing, once it has been discussed with and offered to the patient, the clinician should document the patient's intentions, particularly when multiple providers are caring for the patient. Such documentation will help ensure that proper testing and follow-up on the test results is done.*

3.  The resident, who should have ordered the AFP, was unaware that it was hospital policy for all pregnant women to be offered this test.

    *Clinicians need to be familiar with the policies and procedures of the institutions in which they practice. Orientation should always include review of the applicable policies and procedures and where reference copies are kept.*

4.  At 18 weeks, the radiologist read the ultrasound as normal. A second reading, after the delivery, identified a subtle, but clearly detectable heart defect consistent with Down's syndrome.

    *Improper reading of a test raises concerns regarding the practitioner's skills and the institution's quality. Deviation from standard practice may need to be assessed in an objective manner, by peer review committee. Some institutions put into place systems to help prevent clinicians from missing potentially significant findings, such as double readings of certain radiological tests, in which two clinicians independently review the same films.*

(http://www.rmf.harvard.edu/case-studies)

**Case Study**

**Failure to Respond to Fetal Distress (RN Named as Defendant)**

Upon admission at 10:30 p.m., the patient was placed on an external monitor, and the fetal heart rate was noted to be in the 140's, reactive with good long-term variability. The patient was evaluated by the physician and determined to be in active labor. At 1:45 a.m., the physician documented that the fetal heart rate was in the130's with some variable decelerations, and that the patient was fully dilated. The plan was to have the patient start pushing, and to decrease the epidural pump. According to the plaintiff's expert physician, the fetal monitor tracings from the time of admission until 2:00 a.m. were reactive and reassuring.

At 2:00 a.m., the defendant (the RN) documented that the fetal heart rate was in the 120's, with decelerations to 80-90 with contractions, with slow recovery, and "head stimulation with effect." At 2:30 a.m., the defendant documented that the fetal heart rate was in the 140's with accelerations to 160, and late decelerations to 90-100, with good response to head stimulation. She noted "slow progress with pushing." At 2:50 a.m., the defendant noted that the fetal heart rate baseline increased to 170 at times, and that the IV was infusing wide open. At 3:00 a.m., the defendant initiated a Pitocin drip at 2 mU Per a prior order by the physician. At 3:05 a.m., the defendant documented that the fetal heart tracing showed a baseline of 170-180, with decelerations to 90.

Plaintiff's expert review of the fetal monitor tapes between 2:00a.m. and 3:05 a.m. finds a significant change in the fetal heart tracing. Plaintiff's experts state that there was decreased variability, recurrent decelerations in the fetal heart rate, and a rising fetal heart rate baseline. These findings were non-reassuring and highly suggestive of fetal hypoxia, requiring immediate evaluation by a physician. There is no indication in the medical record that the physician was present in the room between 2:00 a.m. and 3:05 a.m. and the evidence presented during discovery confirmed that the physician was not present and had not been notified of any changes on the monitor during this time frame. During this time, the only intrauterine resuscitative measure noted was a fluid bolus. It was also noted by the plaintiff's attorney, that the defendant made the decision to start a Pitocin infusion in the presence of a non-reassuring fetal heart tracing and without physician evaluation of the tracing.

At 3:15 a.m., the defendant gave a verbal report to the physician. At 3:18 a.m., the physician was noted in the room. Oxygen was administered and the patient was placed on her left side. Special Care Nursery and Pediatrics were summoned, and the patient was prepped for delivery. At 3:51 a.m., the baby was delivered vaginally, weighing 3742 grams (8 lbs. 4 oz.). He was floppy, and without respiratory effort. A loose nuchal cord x2 was present, as well as terminal meconium. His Apgar scores were 2, 6, and 6 and cord pH was 7.24. The baby was intubated, resuscitated, and transferred to the Special Care Nursery. He was later transferred to Children's Hospital.

While at Children's Hospital, he experienced seizure activity and a head CT scan at approximately 9 hours of life showed a small subdural hemorrhage, and brain MRI performed on his first day of life revealed findings consistent with hypoxic/ischemic changes. Additional findings also showed global organ involvement. The baby was diagnosed with cerebral palsy and spastic quadriplegia. He is confined to a wheelchair and he cannot walk, talk or hold his head upright.

During discovery, the defendant argued that the fetal heart rate tracing was reassuring. Prior to trial, the case settled for two million dollars.

(http://www.lubinandmeyer.com/cases/cerebralpalsy

**Telephone Advice**

After a normal delivery, the mother and her newborn baby girl were discharged. A note in the medical record on the day of the discharge stated that the baby had mild diarrhea and jaundice which was considered to be of no significance.

During the first night at home, the baby experienced watery green stools and the following morning the mother called a neighborhood clinic to complain that her baby could not keep any formula down. She expressed concern that something "was definitely wrong." A clinic nurse advised her to change the formula.

The following day, the mother called (call #2) the clinic nurse again to tell her that the change in formula had not improved the baby's diarrhea. The clinic nurse advised her to give the formula "a day or two."

On Day 3, the mother thought the baby looked quite ill. She called the clinic and expressed her concern. The clinic nurse suggested that she bring the baby in to the clinic during walk-in hours that afternoon.

When seen by the clinic nurse, the baby had a high pitched cry, a 101 degree temperature, and appeared dehydrated. The mother and father were advised to take their daughter to a nearby hospital emergency department. The parents drove the baby to the ED themselves as the clinic did not provide or call for emergency transport.

Immediately on arrival to the ED, the baby began to have seizures. She was admitted to the NICU with a primary diagnosis of hypernatremic dehydration. She suffered from intraventricular bleeding and seizures secondary to the dehydration. She presently suffers from spastic quadriplegia and retardation.

Suit was brought against the nurse and parent hospital of the clinic. The case was settled in the high range ($500,000 - $999,999).

Analysis

1. Telephone Advice: the clinic nurse recalled speaking with the mother only one time, concerning diarrhea and formula. She recalled telling the mother to bring the baby to the clinic if the diarrhea continued. However, the phone conversation between the nurse and mother was not documented, since the clinic's policy was to document such conversations when the call was from a patient with an existing medical record.

   *Some documentation in the record about the advice given to the mother may have supported the defense. In this case, systems were not in place to help the provider care for the patient: there was no provision for*

165

*documenting calls except in a patient record, which did not exist in this case. Facilities must have policies and procedures in place, such as log books, to record: the date and time of the call, the name of the caller, the nature of the problem, the advice given, the name of the provider giving the advice, and what advice was given to the caller about procedures to follow if more serious symptoms develop. There should also be a system in place to ensure that an MD regularly reviews all documented calls.*

2. Communication: the record is not clear about whether or not the mother received specific instructions verbal or written, or what to do or who to call if she had questions.

    *The baby was discharged with jaundice, and though the record describes the condition as "not significant," some follow up on the part of the hospital may have been necessary. Clearly, the clinic did not expect her to call with questions and was unacquainted with her situation.*

3. Coordination of Care: when the child was finally seen by the clinic nurse and an emergency department visit was advised, the clinic told the parents to drive the child themselves.

    *This baby was critically ill and emergency transportation should have been obtained.*

(http://www.rmf.harvard.edu/case-studies)

**Case Study**

**Newborn Medication Error**[1]

**Wright v. Abbott Laboratories - D.C. # 97-CV-1333-JTM**

A newborn was transferred to the NICU after being resuscitated in the delivery room. The newborn's blood pressure was checked every 15 minutes and glucose monitoring was performed every hour. A resident was called about the newborn's low blood pressure and ordered "I.V. piggyback normal saline, 20 cc. over 30 minutes". Nurse Karen Diltz overheard Nurse Donna Benjamin repeating the order and asked if she could help. Nurse Diltz did not read the physician's orders (that was recorded by a third nurse, Nurse Rhonda Martin) and relied on what she heard Nurse Benjamin repeating.

Nurse Diltz removed a vial from the medication cart. The cart contained vials of both 0.9% and 14.6% sodium chloride. Nurse Diltz drew 25 cc from the vial of 14.6% sodium chloride and gave the syringe to Nurse Benjamin who injected it into the I.V. line. Less than an hour later, the resident ordered another 20 cc of normal saline. Nurse Diltz used a vial of 14.6% sodium chloride and withdrew 25 cc and gave the syringe to Nurse Benjamin who administered it. The newborn sustained severe permanent physical injuries as the result of the concentrated saline injections. A medical malpractice suit was filed by the parents.

Standards of Care Breached by Nurses Diltz and Benjamin:
Nurse Benjamin was not authorized to administer I.V. medications.
Nurse Diltz:

- ❖ Did not write down the verbal order and READ it back.
- ❖ Knew that a normal saline vial held only 10 cc, yet she drew up 25 cc of concentrated sodium chloride twice from a vial.
- ❖ Did not read the label of the vial containing the concentrated sodium chloride although she testified that it was her normal practice to read it 3 times.
- ❖ Gave the syringe to a nurse who was not authorized to administer its contents.

# Case Studies

## Case Study

## Vague Talk Between OB and RN Caused Delay

A 26-year-old female, G3 P0 AB 2, with a full term uncomplicated pregnancy, experienced pain and leaking fluid. She was unsure if she was in labor, and called her obstetrician, who advised her to use a peri pad, rest, and call back if the symptoms increased. About 2 hours later she went to the ED in severe pain. She was admitted to the Labor and Delivery unit at 8:15 p.m., presenting with leaking green/brown fluid.

The L & D nurse placed her on an electronic fetal monitor (EFM). The patient was 1-2 cm dilated and 50 percent effaced. Per EFM, the fetus was showing heart rate decelerations to 90 bpm and decreased variability. Meconium was present on the patient's peri pad. The patient requested analgesics for pain, and the RN called the obstetrician. She advised him that the EFM strip looked good, and requested an order for Nubain IM for pain, which was administered shortly thereafter.

The obstetrician arrived at 9:20 p.m. Meconium was still present, and the EFM strip showed some decelerations and decreased variability. The obstetrician questioned if it might be due to either the Nubain or to the EFM picking up the maternal pulse. He decided to treat her conservatively with hydration and oxygen. The patient was 3 cm dilated, and she received an epidural.

At 10:50 p.m., as the EFM showed late decelerations and decreased variability, the RN called the obstetrician to the patient's room. The patient was now 5 cm dilated. Fetal scalp pH tests were done by the obstetrician, and results were abnormal at 7.15. The obstetrician determined that the fetus was in distress, and ordered an emergency Cesarean section.

An infant girl was born at 11;24 p.m., weighing 2940 grams, with Apgar scores of 1 at 1 minute, 5 at 5 minutes and 7 at 10 minutes. Her heart rate was less than 80, and she required vigorous resuscitation. Upon admission to the neonatal ICU, the baby's hematocrit was noted to be 12; the retic count was 12.3, and the cord pH was 7.00. A Kleihauer-Betke test revealed significant fetal-maternal bleed. The infant ultimately developed seizures and was diagnosed with hypoxic ischemic encephalopathy. She suffers neurological sequelae from cerebral palsy including right sided hemiparesis, cognitive difficulty and speech delays.

The parents sued the covering obstetrician and the nurse, alleging failure to appropriately assess fetal status and perform a cesarean section in a timely manner.

The case was settled for $1 million.

Analysis

1. The RN did not accurately communicate the maternal-fetal status to the obstetrician, affecting the physician's treatment decisions and causing delay in the diagnosis of fetal distress.

   *When the decision maker is not with the patient, communication from the clinician on site becomes paramount for seeing the whole picture. Specific significant results, such as EFM tracings must be shared during the phone consult. An incomplete status report may lead the physician in charge to miss important clues necessary to understand what is needed next.*

2. Administration of an analgesic (Nubain) without a baseline EFM may have misled the obstetrician, who initially failed to recognize fetal distress, delaying performance of an emergent Cesarean section.

   *New medications initiated at the hospital can complicate ongoing patient evaluation. A normal baseline can offer information as to what is happening in the moment. A non-reassuring baseline gives the physician a potentially critical piece of information about the effects of a new drug and whether to attribute symptoms to something more threatening.*

3. The obstetrician initially told the patient to stay home during her first call.

   *Telephone assessments in a case that is perceived as "low-risk" present a risk of under-evaluation of what the patient is experiencing. Probing questions that a high-risk pregnancy requires may be important for any pregnancy. Instructions must be well understood and well communicated. Prenatal visits should include counseling regarding awareness of danger signs, as well as how to report/communicate those signs to the obstetrician. Good documentation of all phone conversations that have taken place will result in better flow of information and ultimately better care of the patient.*

4. During the RN's call to the obstetrician after her initial assessment of the patient, she did not communicate the abnormal EFM findings or the meconium-stained peri pad.

   *Care teams need to develop an understanding of what needs to be communicated during patient status reports over the telephone. In order to consider more urgent possibilities in the differential diagnosis, all providers must understand the value of their observations. Physicians and nurses can use mental or written checklists to make sure everyone knows about the presence of significant symptoms.*

(http://www.rmf.harvard.edu/case-studies)

Case Studies

**Omissions in Documentation**

**Tammy Derry v. Edward Peskin, MD, Saint Vincent Hospital, Arthur Curtis, MD, Susan Palmer, RN, American Medical Response, Lisa Lavoie, EMT, David Wiggins, EMT (1999)**

Mrs. Derry presented to the emergency department at St. Vincent's hospital in preterm labor. An ultrasound revealed no amniotic fluid and the fetus to be in a breech presentation. Dr. Curtis made the decision to transfer her to another medical facility for management of delivery. The fetal heart rate tracing showed evidence of fetal distress. Despite the fact that the fetus was exhibiting increased fetal heart rate baseline variability, the patient was medicated and discharged to the other facility.

Mrs. Derry arrived at the receiving hospital 50 minutes later. Assessment by ultrasound at this time revealed no amniotic fluid and a fetal heart rate in the 40's. The umbilical cord had prolapsed into the vagina. Mr. and Mrs. Derry were counseled as to the grave prognosis for their unborn baby who was delivered 1 hour and 20 minutes later without a heartbeat.

A law suit was filed and during discovery it was made known that no documentation existed of assessment of Mrs. Derry or her unborn child during transport. To further complicate the case, several consent forms were either missing from the chart or were present but not signed. The case was not able to be defended.

Source: Helm, A. (2003). Nursing Malpractice: Sidestepping Legal Minefields. Lippincott: Philadelphia.

**Case Study**

**Failure to Assess and Intervene**

**Baptist Medical Center Montclair v. Wilson (1993)**

The patient, a VBAC candidate, was admitted to the labor and delivery unit in early labor. Hours later the patient experienced a sharp pain in her abdomen. Within moments the patient and her husband noticed vaginal bleeding. The patient told the nurse she felt as though her stomach had ripped open and the baby had moved up toward the ceiling. Approximately 20 minutes later, the nurse performed a cervical exam and determined the patient's cervix was completely dilated. The fetal heart had dropped to 60 beats per minute. The nurse then notified the physician of her assessment, but did not report the sharp abdominal pain. Fifteen minutes later the physician examined the patient. And found she was not dilated. An emergency cesarean section delivery followed. The delivery occurred almost one hour following the patient's report of abdominal pain. The patient had suffered a uterine rupture. Fetal distress resulted as the baby was pushed into the abdominal cavity causing placental abruption. The infant died at 5 months of age.

Deviations from the Standard of Care That Were Noted at Trial - Failure To:
- Notify the physician of the sharp abdominal pain
- Carry out intrauterine resuscitative measures
- Properly and completely assess the patient

Case Studies

## Case Study

## Failure to Assess and Intervene

## Province v. Center for Women's Health and Family Birth (1993)

The patient notified the nurse that she felt something "like a heartbeat in my vagina" and that it was "pulsating". The patient also asked the nurse to call her doctor, but the nurse did not because she felt the complaint was insignificant.

The patient was later permitted to ambulate to the restroom where she noticed the umbilical cord protruding. An emergency section was performed, but the infant suffered severe brain damage.

**Case Study**

**Failure to Interpret Fetal Distress**

**Fairfax Hospital System, Inc. v McCarty (1992)**

Mrs. McCarty was 31 years old when she was admitted to Fairfax Hospital to deliver her first child. Mrs. McCarty was placed on an electronic fetal monitor at about 7:30 A.M. after spontaneous rupture of membranes. A nurse began attending to her about 6:10 P.M. that evening and was to be with her until 9:00 P.M. The evidence presented in court established that the fetal heart rate monitor demonstrated a broad-based deceleration at approximately 8:27 P.M. The mother began demonstrating an abnormal labor pattern and the fetal heart rate monitor demonstrated that the fetus was experiencing more and more difficulty. In spite of the fetal distress apparent on the fetal monitor strip as early as 8:27 P.M., the nurse did not notify the physician until 8:50 P.M.

The obstetrician, testifying for the plaintiffs, indicated that the nurse did not tell him an emergency situation was present. He testified that a cesarean delivery could have been accomplished within 12 minutes and that had he seen the fetal monitor, he would have moved to deliver the infant shortly before 8:40 P.M. The obstetrician further testified that the nurse's failure to take action or notify him delayed delivery and contributed to the eventual outcome of the infant. The infant has severe neurological impairments.

Settlement: $3.5 million dollars.

Case Studies

**Case Study**

**Telephone Triage**

**Descheness v. Anonymous (1992)**

A gravida 3 para1 female delivered following a prolonged second stage of labor. The obstetrician performed a Scanzoni maneuver which involved the rotation of the baby's head with mid forceps. The delivery was then accomplished with the assistance of low forceps. The mother experienced abdominal pain and difficulty urinating during the postpartum period.

During the next several days she reported by phone to the office that she was experiencing severe pain, hardening of her abdomen, cramps, nausea, fever, fatigue, and seepage from her vagina. These symptoms were attributed to flu and constipation but the patient was not seen for examination. Nine days after birth, she was taken to the hospital. The woman was diagnosed with sepsis, ARDS, and a perforated bladder. She died several days later. Few records of the calls were produced with only one doctor admitting to speaking with the patient.

Settlement: $1.3 million dollars.

**Case Study**

**Nurses Exonerated Based on Documentation and Assessment of Patient**

**Pugh v. Mayeaux, 702 S. 2d 988 (La.App. 1998)**

At full term, Mrs. Pugh was admitted to the hospital with intermittent labor contractions and slight cervical dilation. Shortly after her admission, the nurse noted that Mrs. Pugh showed signs of possible pancreatitis. The nurse called the physician and received orders for continuous fetal monitoring for signs of fetal distress and to be notified should the fetus show signs of distress.

According to the medical record, nurses assessed Mrs. Pugh 10 times between 1500 and 2315. At 1616, the physician called to prescribe an antiemetic in response to a nurse's report that Mrs. Pugh continued to have mild nausea and emesis. At 2315, the nurse telephoned the physician to report that the patient had abdominal distention and diffuse abdominal pain, was vomiting dark green emesis, and had a temperature of 99.3 degrees. The physician ordered a STAT amylase level and insertion of a nasogastric tube connected to continuous low suction. The nurse implemented these orders.

When the laboratory results showed an above-normal amylase level, suggesting pancreatitis, the nurse called the physician again. He decided not to perform an emergency cesarean section because the pancreatitis did not threaten the fetus. He also ordered continuous fetal monitoring and instructed the nurse to contact him immediately if she detected signs of fetal distress.

At 0445 the next day, the nurse telephoned the physician to report that Mrs. Pugh had continuing abdominal distress and distention. She was taken to the intensive care unit. Later that morning, when the fetal heart rate dropped, the nurse notified the physician immediately and prepared the patient for a cesarean section.

An emergency cesarean section was performed, but the baby had hypoxic neurologic damage. The parents sued the doctor, nurses and hospital for negligence in not performing the cesarean section sooner.

The court exonerated the defendants. It found that the nurses had provided high quality care and documented their care thoroughly, as shown by their notes describing comprehensive assessment, prompt physician notification of assessment data, and immediate implementation of the physician's orders.

Source: Surefire Documentation: How What, and When Nurses Need to Document (1999). Goldberg, K. (Ed). Mosby: Philadelphia.

Case Studies

**Criminal Complaint Filed Against Nurse**

**State of Wisconsin**

**Case No. 2006 CF 2512**

Summary of the report filed by Gregory Schuler, an investigator with the Wisconsin Department of Justice, Medicaid Fraud Control Unit (MFCU). The MFCU is charged with investigating and prosecuting criminal offenses affecting the medical assistance program, including laws affecting health, safety, and welfare of recipients of medical assistance.

On July 5, 2006, Jasmine Gant (age 16) was admitted to Saint Mary's Medical Center, Madison, Wisconsin, in labor. No identification bracelet was placed on Ms. Gant. Due to a strep throat, the patient was to receive Penicillin. The nurse stated that she decided to get a bag of Bupivacaine from the Pyxis to show the patient and placed it on the counter. Contrary to what others in the room reported, the defendant RN insisted that Ms. Gant began "crying" and was in a "panic" causing the defendant to inadvertently pick up the bag of Bupivacaine instead of the Penicillin which another nurse had placed on the counter.

The nurse admitted that she did not look at the bag and that she was not planning to scan the medication in the Bridge System until after she administered the medication (clearly defeating the purpose of scanning). Within five minutes of receiving the Bupivacaine IV, Ms. Gant experienced a seizure, was gasping for air and clenching her jaw. She was declared dead at 18:30.

The report cited that the defendant RN failed to:

- Place an identification bracelet on the patient upon admission.
- Obtain authorization to remove the lethal chemicals that caused the patient's death from a locked storage system (the Pyxis). Epidural anesthesia had not been ordered.
- Scan the bar code on the medication, a process of which the defendant had been fully trained and cognizant of.
- Read the bright, clearly written warning on the bag containing the Bupivacaine.
- Follow the approved rate for any medication that may have been ordered, in an apparent effort to save time. The rapid introduction of these chemicals dramatically hastened the death of the patient.
- Follow the "five rights "of medication administration.

This was a class H Felony which carried the maximum penalty of a fine not to exceed $25,000 or imprisonment not to exceed 6 years, or both.

## Medication Error Leads to Indictment for Criminally Negligent Homicide

### The Denver Case

During prenatal care, the patient was found to have a positive Rapid Plasma Reagin (RPR). When questioned, the patient reported having contracted syphilis in 1981 and that it had been treated at that time. The Colorado State Health Department attempted to verify the 1981 treatment, but was unable to confirm that treatment had been provided. The obstetrician chose not to treat the patient though CDC guidelines recommend that patients be treated. RPR titers were repeated at 18 and 29 weeks and were noted to be positive. At 36 weeks the antepartum record was sent to the hospital. A titer was drawn at 38 weeks and the result was negative, but not communicated to the hospital.[2]

The patient was delivered at 40 weeks and the neonatologist chose to treat the newborn since he was not aware of the negative results. Benzathine Penicillin G IM was ordered. The dose was to be 150,000 units. However, the pharmacist filled the physician's order with 10 times the ordered dose and a pre-filled 2.5 ml syringe with 1,500,000 units was sent to the nursery. The nurse was concerned that the baby would need multiple injections due to the large volume, but did not call the pharmacy to verify the dose and instead decided to administer the medication IV. The NNP believed the Benzathine to be a brand name for Penicillin (it is actually the solution in which the Penicillin is suspended and Aqueous is the proper intravenous medium). The NNP and nursery nurse administered the medication IV and the baby arrested within 3 minutes and was not able to be revived.

Aftermath of this tragic error:
- The NNP was terminated and the nursery nurse was assigned non-nursing duties; both had their licenses suspended for a period of time
- The pharmacist was allowed to resign, reported to the State Board of Pharmacy, investigated, but not disciplined.
- The District Attorney investigated the case and the NNP, nursery nurse and nurse assigned to care for the mother and baby were indicted in the criminal court on charges of negligent homicide (reckless and wanton disregard for life).
- Several days before the trial, the NNP and nursery nurse decided to accept a plea bargain. According to the agreement, the nurses' records would be expunged of the conviction provided they avoid any further criminal convictions for two years. The plea bargain removed the immediate possibility of a prison sentence and/or fines for both of the nurses.[2]
- The baby's nurse chose to go to trial and was acquitted on January 30, 1998.

177

Multiple errors were identified in this case:[2]

➤ Inadequate documentation of the plan of care regarding the patient's treatment for syphilis.

➤ Lack of communication between the obstetrician and neonatologist.

➤ Language barrier (the patient spoke Spanish) which was thought to precipitate the need for immediate treatment.

➤ The pharmacist made a serious error in interpreting the physician's order.

➤ The nurses did not question the large volume of medication sent to the nursery.

➤ The 5 rights of medication administration were not followed. The NNP and nurse lacked experience administering the medication but did not seek advice.

➤ There were no written protocols at this institution for neonatal nurse practitioners.

1. Helm A. *Nursing Malpractice: Sidestepping Legal Minefields.* Philadelphia: Lippincott, Williams & Wilkins; 2003.
2. Kowalski K, Horner MD. A legal nightmare. Denver nurses indicted. *MCN Am J Matern Child Nurs.* 1998; 23:125-129.

# Additional Resources

## to Supplement the Books and Articles Previously Referenced

**List of Additional Resources and Websites**

**Academy of Certified Birth Educators and Labor Support Professionals (ACBE)**
http://www.acbe.com

**Agency for Healthcare Research and Quality (AHRQ)**
http://www.ahrq.gov
AHRQ is the lead federal agency in supporting and implementing the recommendations of the IOM in its effort to reduce medical error and improve patient safety. The Agency for Healthcare Research and Quality (AHRQ) website has extensive resources in its "Quality and Patient Safety Section." The AHRQ website also provides access to the Patient Safety Indicators (PSIs), a tool to help health system leaders identify potential in-hospital complications and adverse events following surgeries, procedures, and childbirth. (For more information on PSIs, see http://www.qualityindicators.ahrq.gov/psi_overview.htm)

**American Academy of Pediatrics (AAP)**
http://www.aap.org

**American Association of Critical Care Nurses (AACN)**
http://www.aacn.org

**American Association of Legal Nurse Consultants (AALNC)**
http://www.aalnc.org
Founded in 1989, the American Association of Legal Nurse Consultants (AALNC) is a not for profit membership organization dedicated to the professional enhancement and growth of registered nurses practicing in the specialty area of legal nurse consulting and to advancing this nursing specialty.

**American Bar Association (ABA)**
http://www.abanet.org
Referral to an attorney; client's rights and responsibilities; information about preventing and resolving common problems with your attorney.

# Additional Resources

## American College of Obstetricians and Gynecologists (ACOG)

http://www.acog.org

## American College of Nurse Midwives (ACNM)

http://www.acnm.org

## American Health Information Management Association (AHIMA)

http://www.ahima.org

AHIMA is the premier association of health information management (HIM) professionals. AHIMA's 52,000 members are dedicated to the effective management of personal health information needed to deliver quality healthcare to the public. Founded in 1928 to improve the quality of medical records, AHIMA is committed to advancing the HIM profession in an increasingly electronic and global environment through leadership in advocacy, education, certification, and lifelong learning.

## American Nurses Association (ANA)

http://www.ana.org

## American Nurses Credentialing Center (ANCC)

http://www.ana.org

The American Nurses Credentialing Center (ANCC), a subsidiary of the American Nurses Association (ANA), provides individuals and organizations throughout the nursing profession with the resources they need to achieve practice excellence. ANCC's internationally renowned credentialing programs certify nurses in specialty practice areas; recognize healthcare organizations for promoting safe, positive work environments through the Magnet Recognition Program® and the Pathway to Excellence Program™ and accredit providers of continuing nursing education. In addition, ANCC provides leading-edge information and education services and products to support its core credentialing programs.

## American Society for Healthcare Risk Management (ASHRM)

http://www.ashrm.org

The ASHRM Foundation was developed to help facilitate the advancement of the risk management profession by funding education, scholarships and research programs. The mission of the Foundation is to secure resources and administer assets (including informational materials) that provide support for meeting ASHRM's strategic goals in education and research.

## Association of Women's Health, Obstetric and Neonatal Nurses (AWHONN)

http://www.awhonn.org

The Association of Women's Health, Obstetric and Neonatal Nurses (AWHONN) is a 501(c)3 nonprofit membership organization that promotes the health of women and newborns. Their mission is to improve and promote the health of women and newborns and to strengthen the nursing profession through the delivery of superior advocacy, research, education and other professional and clinical resources to nurses and other health care professionals.

## Centers for Disease Control and Prevention (CDC)

http://www.cdc.gov

## Center for Medical Simulation

www.harvardmedsim.org

The Center for Medical Simulation (CMS) focuses on improving patient safety and healthcare quality by using simulation for education, training and research. The Center's programs focus on communication, collaboration and crisis management to develop skills and behaviors that are best learned actively under realistic conditions to improve performance of individuals and teams in the real world.

## Cochrane Database of Systematic Reviews

http://www.cochrane.com

The Cochrane Library contains high-quality, independent evidence to inform healthcare decision-making. It includes reliable evidence from Cochrane and other systematic reviews, clinical trials, and more. Cochrane reviews bring you the combined results of the world's best medical research studies, and are recognized as the gold standard in evidence-based health care.

## Institute for Healthcare Improvement (IHI)

http://www.ihi.org

The Institute for Healthcare Improvement (IHI) is an independent not-for-profit organization helping to lead the improvement of health care throughout the world. Founded in 1991 and based in Cambridge, Massachusetts, IHI works to accelerate improvement by building the will for change, cultivating promising concepts for improving patient care, and helping health care systems put those ideas into action.

## Institute for Safe Medication Practices

http://www.ismp.org

The Institute for Safe Medication Practices (ISMP) "Pathways for Medication Safety: Leading a Strategic Planning Effort" tool can assist senior leaders in assessing the current status of medication safety in their organizations to develop a strategic plan for moving forward (see http://www.ismp.org/PDF/PathwaySection1.pdf). The "2004 ISMP Medication Safety Self-Assessment for Hospitals" is a self-assessment tool that examines key elements in the hospital that influence safe medication use (see http://www.ismp.org/selfassessments/Hospital/2004Hospsm.pdf)

## International Board of Lactation Consultant Examiners (IBLCE)

http://www.nursingcenter.com

## International Childbirth Education Association (ICEA)

http://www.icea.org

## Joint Commission on Accreditation of Healthcare Organizations (JCAHO)

http://www.jcaho.org

The Joint Commission evaluates and accredits more than 15,000 health care organizations and programs in the United States. An independent, not-for-profit organization, The Joint Commission is the nation's predominant standards-setting and accrediting body in health care. Its mission is to continuously improve the safety and quality of care provided to the public through the provision of health care accreditation and related services that support performance improvement in health care organizations.

## Joint Commission International Center for Patient Safety

http://www.jcipatientsafety.org/

This website provides resources and information about patient safety for patients and their families, as well as health care professionals, including physicians, nurses, pharmacists, and other allied professionals. The Joint Commission's National Patient Safety Goals can be accessed via the website, along with timely Sentinel Event Alerts.

## Journal of Patient Safety

http://www.journalpatientsafety.com

Journal of Patient Safety is dedicated to presenting research advances and field applications in every area of patient safety. While Journal of Patient Safety has a research emphasis, it also publishes articles describing near-miss opportunities, system modifications that are barriers to error, and the impact of regulatory changes on healthcare delivery.

## Lamaze Childbirth Educator Certification (LCEC)

http://www.lamaze-childbirth.com

## March of Dimes (MOD)

http://www.modimes.org

## National Association of Neonatal Nurses (NANN)

http://www.nann.org

## National Certification Corporation for the Obstetric, Gynecologic and Neonatal Specialties (NCC)

http://www.nccnet.org

The National Certification Corporation (NCC) is a not for profit organization that provides a national credentialing program for nurses, physicians and other licensed health care personnel. Certification is awarded to nurses in the obstetric, gynecologic, neonatal and telephone nursing specialties and certificates of added qualification are awarded in the subspecialty areas of electronic fetal monitoring, breastfeeding, gynecologic health care and menopause

## National Council of State Boards of Nursing

http://www.ncsbn.org

Information about the nurse practice act, misconduct laws, and disciplinary processes in your state: keeps a data base of nurses who have been disciplined.

## National Guideline Clearing House
http://www.guideline.gov

The National Guideline Clearinghouse™ (NGC) is a comprehensive database of evidence-based clinical practice guidelines and related documents. NGC is an initiative of the Agency for Healthcare Research and Quality (AHRQ), U.S. Department of Health and Human Services. NGC was originally created by AHRQ in partnership with the American Medical Association and the American Association of Health Plans (now America's Health Insurance Plans [AHIP]). The NGC mission is to provide physicians, nurses, and other health professionals, health care providers, health plans, integrated delivery systems, purchasers and others an accessible mechanism for obtaining objective, detailed information on clinical practice guidelines and to further their dissemination, implementation and use.

## National Patient Safety Foundation (NPSF)
http://www.npsf.org

## National Quality Forum
http://www.qualityforum.org/

The National Quality Forum (NQF) is a not-for-profit membership organization created to develop and implement a national strategy for health care quality measurement and reporting. In 2003 NQF published "Safe Practices for Better Healthcare," a consensus report that identified 30 health care safe practices and recommended that all applicable health care settings implement these practices to reduce the risk of harm to patients. (For more information on the report, see http://www.quality forum.org/txsafeexecsumm+order6-8-03PUBLIC.pdf)

## Nurse Advocate
http://www.nurseadvocate.org

Information and E-mail list related to workplace violence, including abuse, harassment, and horizontal violence.

## Nurse Protect, Inc.
http://www.nurseprotect.com

Referral to an attorney with a reputation for successful representation of nurses; information about misconduct, discipline, and the disciplinary climate in your state; peer support is available.

**Peri-FACTS**

http://www.urmc.edu/obgyn/Peri-FACTS

Peri-FACTS is a weekly, multimedia eJournal program that provides ongoing, quality, continuing education to obstetric care providers across the nation and abroad. Distributed directly to subscribers via the Internet, it provides up-to-date information on obstetric issues that are most commonly encountered in the United States. Utilizing a combination of clinical case studies and didactic reading materials, Peri-FACTS teaches the principles of fetal heart monitoring and general obstetric care.

**Risk Management Foundation (RMF)**

http://www.rmf.harvard.edu

Risk Management Foundation (RMF) was incorporated by the Harvard Medical Institutions in 1979 as a charitable, medical and educational membership organization. Today, CRICO/RMF is an internationally renowned leader in evidence-based risk management. It serves nearly 10,000 physicians, 18 hospitals, and 238 other healthcare organizations.

**State Nurses Association**

http://www.nursingworld.org/snaweb.htm

Lists of attorneys with a proven track record representing nurses; information about misconduct, discipline, and the disciplinary climate in your state; peer support.

**The Leapfrog Group**

http://www.leapfroggroup.org/for_hospitals

The Leapfrog Group is a voluntary initiative in which organizations that buy health care are working together to initiate breakthrough improvements in the safety, quality, and affordability of health care for Americans. The Leapfrog Group has several patient safety resources for hospitals, including research and selected references on Computerized Physician Order Entry (CPOE) systems.

**United States Food and Drug Administration (FDA)**

http://www.fda.gov

# Fetal Heart Monitoring

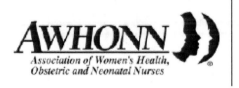

## AWHONN Clinical Position Statement

AWHONN supports the assessment of the laboring woman and her fetus during labor through the use of auscultation, palpation and/or electronic fetal monitoring (EFM) techniques. The availability of registered nurses and other health care professionals who are skilled in maternal-fetal assessment, to include fetal heart monitoring (FHM) techniques is important for optimal care of the mother and her fetus. AWHONN recognizes that the fetal auscultation and palpation of uterine activity as well as the judicious application of intrapartum EFM are appropriate and effective methods to assess and promote maternal and fetal well-being. Current research indicates that fetal heart rate auscultation, when provided with a 1:1 nurse-patient ratio, is comparable to EFM for fetal assessment of the laboring woman. It is important that a woman's preference be taken into account whenever possible when deciding on FHM techniques.

Fetal heart monitoring requires advanced assessment and clinical judgment skills, regardless of the setting in which it is used. Therefore, each aspect of FHM should be performed by licensed, experienced health care professionals consistent with their state or provincial scope of practice. AWHONN maintains that fetal heart monitoring (FHM) includes:
- application of fetal monitoring components;
- intermittent auscultation;
- ongoing monitoring and interpretation of FHM data;
- initial assessment of the laboring woman and fetus; and
- ongoing clinical interventions and evaluations of the woman and fetus.

Initiation of monitoring and ongoing clinical evaluation should only be performed by health care professionals who have education and skills validation in FHM and in the care of the laboring woman. AWHONN regards these health care professionals with expertise in fetal monitoring as:
- registered nurses;
- certified nurse midwives (CNMs), certified midwives (CMs) and registered midwives (RMs-Canada);
- other advanced practice nurses such as nurse practitioners and clinical

  nurse specialists;
- physicians; and
- physician assistants

AWHONN believes fetal heart monitoring should not be delegated to other personnel who do not possess this level of licensure, education, and skill validation.

AWHONN does not support the use of EFM as a substitute for appropriate professional nursing care and support of women in labor. Facilities should ensure registered nurse staffing levels that meet the changing needs and acuity of the laboring woman and her fetus throughout the intrapartum period. Facilities should incorporate relevant recommendations from professional associations and organizations, and state, federal and/or provincial regulations into FHM policies and procedures.

AWHONN recommends a 1:1 nurse-to-patient ratio during the second stage of labor because of the nature and intensity of care required during this period. This staffing ratio should be maintained whether EFM or auscultation and palpation are used to assess the fetal heart rate and uterine activity.

AWHONN recommends ongoing education and periodic competence validation for registered nurses and other health care professionals who engage in fetal heart monitoring (FHM). To prepare clinicians for the use of auscultation and EFM and the evaluation of uterine activity, AWHONN urges facilities to establish or make available educational programs for guided clinical experiences, skills validation and ongoing competence assessment. AWHONN supports education that includes physiologic interpretation of FHM data, implications for labor support, and interprofessional communication strategies.

Communication and collaboration are essential and central to providing quality care and optimizing patient outcomes. AWHONN supports the need for institutional policies, procedures and protocols that promote collegiality among health care professionals. Many perinatal units have developed excellent professional communication strategies that foster collaborative relationships. However, differences of opinion about professional judgment and decision making related to fetal heart monitoring may occur.

Facilities should establish and maintain interprofessional policies and procedures that allow the registered nurse to make decisions regarding fetal monitoring practice and that identify the appropriate mechanisms to use if there is a difference of opinion in the interpretation of the fetal monitoring data or patient plan of care. These policies should clearly describe the facility chain of authority (also referred to as chain of command) and reflect state, territorial and/or provincial regulations; and consider the recommendations of professional organizations and credentialing bodies. The chain of authority should be present and used to safeguard the best interests of the woman and her baby as well as all members of the health care team.

AWHONN supports organizations' development of a culture of safety as described in recommendations of accrediting bodies and other professional organizations. Research suggests that lack of teamwork is associated with less optimal patient outcomes. Policies, procedures and guidelines should address collegial communication, timely and complete documentation, risk management strategies and staffing appropriate for the clinical needs of the laboring woman and her fetus.

Maternal and fetal clinical information should be documented throughout the course of labor. AWHONN supports the development of interprofessional institutional policies, procedures and protocols that outline responsibility for ongoing fetal heart monitoring (FHM) documentation. Documentation should contain streamlined, factual and objective information and should include, but may not be limited to:
- a systematic admission assessment of the woman and fetus;
- ongoing assessments of the woman and fetus;
- interventions provided and evaluation of responses,
- communication with women and their families or primary support persons;
- communication with providers; and
- communication within the chain of authority.

Ideally, all providers should develop consistent FHM policies that specify the standardized FHM language to be used in a given facility. Registered nurses should use standardized descriptive terms to communicate and document fetal heart rate characteristics (e.g. variability, decelerations, and accelerations). It is within the scope of practice of the nurse to implement customary interventions in response to EFM data and clinical assessment.

AWHONN recommends that institutions clearly delineate the nature of documentation, including style, format, and frequency interval. Documentation does not necessarily need to occur at the same intervals as assessment when utilizing continuous EFM. AWHONN supports the use of summary documentation at intervals established by the individual facility and described within policies, procedures and guidelines. This documentation policy should be based on state and/or provincial guidelines as well as those of professional associations, regulatory and certifying bodies. Each institution should also determine policies and procedures regarding maintenance, storage, archiving and retrieval of all forms of fetal heart monitoring records as well as the parameters of maintaining the FHM tracing as part of the medical record.

AWHONN supports research focused on enhancing the body of knowledge and best practices regarding fetal assessment. Specifically, AWHONN supports research concerning the:

- efficacy of FHM that includes standardized definitions and FHM terminology;
- efficacy of interventions used in response to fetal monitoring findings;
- effect of uterine activity on fetal oxygenation;
- efficacy of EFM related to neonatal outcomes;
- impact of EFM on a woman's labor experience and maternal outcomes;
- impact of staffing on optimal patient outcomes related to fetal assessment and intervention;
- identification of optimal information technology applications; and
- comparisons of patient outcomes and quality indicators when using auscultation and palpation versus EFM.

AWHONN supports policies that promote:

- Promulgation and broad professional acceptance of unified terminology for description and documentation of FHM;
- Consensus regarding interpretation and management of EFM; development of standardized FHM terminology across disciplines;
- Clarity and consensus development among professional organizations and regulatory bodies regarding the scope of practice of licensed health care providers related to the use of FHM.

**Background**

The background section of this position statement has been expanded to provide resource information for clinicians. AWHONN utilizes a variety of publications to promulgate policy and clinical recommendations. AWHONN has done extensive work in the area of fetal heart monitoring. Clinical recommendations are updated on an ongoing basis to keep pace with the current research and practice recommendations that are discussed and promoted by national professional and regulatory organizations. The role of this AWHONN position statement is to articulate the position of the organization on key policy issues within the field of fetal heart monitoring. Clinical recommendations are found in a number of key publications published by AWHONN and other organizations. Selected key publications are noted at the end of this document in Resources.

Two specific clinical recommendations are presented as background for this position statement – frequency of auscultation and fetal assessment in labor. AWHONN encourages practitioners to utilize the full range of fetal heart monitoring resources published.

**Frequency of Assessments in Labor**

**Frequency of Fetal Heart Rate by Auscultation**

Professional associations including the Association of Women's Health, Obstetric and Neonatal Nurses (AWHONN), the American Academy of Pediatrics (AAP) and American College of Obstetricians and Gynecologists (ACOG) (AAP & ACOG, 2007), the Society of Obstetricians and Gynaecologists of Canada (SOGC, 2007), and the Royal College of Obstetricians and Gynaecologists (RCOG, 2001) have suggested protocols for the frequency of assessment of the fetal heart rate by auscultation to determine fetal status during labor. The suggested frequencies are typically based on protocols reported in seminal research clinical trials that compared perinatal outcomes associated with fetal heart rate auscultation and electronic fetal monitoring (Haverkamp, et al., 1979; Haverkamp, Thompson, McFee, & Cetrulo 1976; Kelso, et al., 1978; Luthy, et al. 1987; McDonald, Grant, Sheridan-Pereira, Boylan, & Chalmers, 1985; Neldam, et al., 1986; Renou, Chang, Anderson, & Wood, 1976; Vintzileos et al., 1993). The range of frequency of assessment using auscultation in these studies varied from every 15 – 30 minutes during the active phase of the first stage of labor to every 5-15 minutes during the second stage of labor. In most studies, a 1:1 nurse to patient ratio was used for auscultation protocols. These classic studies included low risk and/or high risk patient populations.

Because variation exists in the original research protocols, clinicians should make decisions about the method and frequency of fetal assessment based on evaluation of factors including patient preferences, the phase and stage of labor, maternal response to labor, assessment of maternal-fetal condition and risk factors, unit staffing resources and facility rules and procedures.

Considering these factors, the suggested frequencies for fetal heart rate auscultation are within the range of every 15 - 30 minutes during the active phase of the first stage of labor and every 5-15 minutes during the active pushing phase of the second stage of labor. No clinical trials have examined fetal surveillance methods during the latent phase of labor. Therefore, health-care providers should use their clinical judgment when deciding the method and frequency of fetal surveillance.

**Frequency of Fetal Assessment with Electronic Fetal Monitoring**
   **In the absence of risk factors:**
            Determine and evaluate the FHR every 30 minutes during the active phase of the first stage of labor and every 15 minutes during the (active pushing phase) of the second stage of labor (AAP & ACOG, 2007). In Canada, the FHR is evaluated every 5 minutes in the active phase of the second stage of labor (SOGC, 2007).
   **When risk factors are present, continuous EFM is recommended:**
            During the active phase of the first stage of labor, the FHR should be determined and evaluated every 15 minutes (AAP & ACOG, 2007). During the active pushing phase of the second stage of labor, the FHR should be determined and evaluated at least every 5 minutes (AWHONN, 2008).

During oxytocin induction or augmentation, the FHR should be determined and evaluated every 15 minutes during the active phase of the first stage of labor and every 5 minutes during the (active pushing phase) of the second stage of labor (AAP & ACOG, 2007; AWHONN 2008).

When EFM is used to record FHR data permanently, periodic documentation can be used to summarize evaluation of fetal status at the frequencies recommended by AAP and ACOG (2007) as outlined by institutional protocols. Thus, while evaluation of the FHR may be occurring every 15 minutes, a summary note including findings of fetal status may be documented in the medical record less frequently. During oxytocin induction or augmentation, the FHR should be evaluated and documented before each dose increase. During the active pushing phase of the second stage of labor, summary documentation of fetal status approximately every 30 minutes indicating there was continuous nursing bedside attendance and evaluation seems reasonable (Simpson, 2008b).

*Approved by the AWHONN Board of Directors, 1988; revised 1992; reaffirmed 1994; revised and re-titled 2000; revised and re-titled November 2008.*

## Resources

American Academy of Pediatrics and American College of Obstetricians and Gynecologists (2007). *Guidelines for Perinatal Care,* 6th ed.): Elk Grove Village, IL: Author.

American College of Obstetricians and Gynecologists. (2005). *Intrapartum fetal heart rate monitoring* (ACOG Practice Bulletin No. 62). Washington, DC: Author.

Simpson, K.R. (2008). *Cervical Ripening and Induction and Augmentation of Labor* (3rd ed.). Washington, DC: Association of Women's Health, Obstetric and Neonatal Nurses (AWHONN).

Association of Women's Health, Obstetric and Neonatal Nurses (2008). *Nursing Care and Management of the Second Stage of Labor,* (2nd ed.). Washington, DC: Author.

Feinstein, N.F., Sprague, A. & Trepanier, M.J. (2008). *Fetal Heart Rate Auscultation* (2nd ed.). Washington DC: Association of Women's Health, Obstetric and Neonatal Nurses (AWHONN)

Joint Commission on Accreditation of Healthcare Organizations (2004). *Preventing infant death and injury during delivery.* (Sentinel Event Alert No. 30.). Oak Brook, IL.

Lyndon, A., & Ali, L. U. (Eds.). (In press). *Fetal Heart Monitoring: Principles and Practices* (4th ed.). Dubuque, IA: Kendall Hunt Publishing.

Society of Obstetricians and Gynaecologists of Canada (SOGC) (2007). Fetal health surveillance: Antepartum and intrapartum consensus guideline. *Journal of Obstetrics and Gynaecology Canada,* 29(9), Supplement 4, S1-S56.

## References

American Academy of Pediatrics and American College of Obstetricians and Gynecologists (2007). *Guidelines for Perinatal Care*, (6th ed.): Elk Grove Village, IL: Author.

Haverkamp, A., Orleans, M., Langendoerfer, S., McFee, J., Murphy, J., & Thompson, H. (1979). A controlled trial of the differential effects of intrapartum fetal monitoring. *American Journal of Obstetrics and Gynecology*, 134, 399-412.

Haverkamp, A., Thompson, H., McFee, J., & Certulo, C. (1976). The evaluation of continuous fetal heart rate monitoring in high-risk pregnancy. *American Journal of Obstetrics and Gynecology*, 125(3). 310-320.

Kelso, I., Parsons, R., Lawrence, G., Arora, S., Edmonds, D., & Cooke, I. (1978). An assessment of continous fetal hear rate monitoring in labor: A randomized trial. *American Journal of Obstetrics & Gynecology*, 131, 526-532.

Luthy, D. A., Shy, K. K., van Belle, G., Larson, E., Hughes, J., Benedetti, T., Brown, Z., Effer, J., King, J., & Stenchever, M. (1987). A randomized trial of electronic fetal monitoring in preterm labor. *Obstetrics & Gynecology*, 69(5), 687-695.

McDonald, D., Grant, A., Sheridan-Pereira, M., Boylan, P., & Chalmers, I. (1985). The Dublin randomized controlled trial of intrapartum fetal heart rate monitoring. *American Journal of Obstetrics & Gynecology*, 152, 524-539.

Neldam, S., Osler, M., Kern Hansen, P., Nim, J., Friis Smith, S., & Hertel, J. (1986). Intrapartum fetal heart rate monitoring in a combined low- and high-risk population: A controlled clinical trial. *European Journal of Obstetrics, Gynecology, and Reproductive Biology*, 23, 1–11.

Renou, P., Chang, A., Anderson, I., & Wood, C. (1976). Controlled trial of fetal intensive care. *American Journal of Obstetrics and Gynecology*, 126(4), 470-475.

Royal College of Obstetricians and Gynaecologists. (2001). *The use of electronic fetal monitoring. The use and interpretation of cardiotocography in intrapartum fetal surveillance.* (Evidence-based Clinical Guideline No. 8). Retrieved November 7, 2008 from http://www.rcog.org.uk/resources/public/pdf/efm_guideline_final_2may2001.pdf.

Simpson, K. R. (2008). Labor and birth. In K. R. Simpson & P. A. Creehan (Eds.), *AWHONN's Perinatal Nursing* (3rd ed., pp 300–398). Philadelphia: Lippincott Williams and Wilkins.

Society of Obstetricians and Gynaecologists of Canada (SOGC). (2007). Fetal Health Surveillance: Antepartum and Intrapartum Consensus Guideline. *Journal of Obstetrics and Gynaecology Canada,* 29(9), Supplement 4, S1-S56.

Thacker, S. B., Stroup, D. F., & Chang, M. (2004). Continuous electronic fetal monitoring for fetal assessment during labor. *Cochrane Database of Systematic Reviews,* Volume 3, Retrieved December 8, 2008 from Ovid Technologies.

Association of Women's Health, Obstetric and Neonatal Nurses
2000 L Street, NW  Suite 740 • Washington, D.C.  20036
202/261-2400 • Fax 202/728-0575 • Canadian 800/245-0231
www.awhonn.org

# The Role of Unlicensed Assistive Personnel in the Nursing Care for Women and Newborns

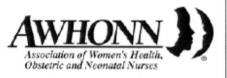

**AWHONN Clinical Position Statement**

The professional registered nurse is the primary nursing care giver and is critical to achieving the most optimal outcomes for women and newborns. AWHONN recognizes that unlicensed assistive personnel (UAPS) can contribute as members of the healthcare team under the direction of the professional registered nurse, who is ultimately responsible for the coordination and delivery of nursing care to women and newborns.

**Background**: When UAPs participate in direct care, the professional registered nurse is the primary nursing care giver and is critical to achieving the most optimal outcomes for women and newborns. When UAPs participate in direct care, parameters for training and supervising these nursing support personnel must be in place. Parameters should include:

- Defining UAPs as unlicensed personnel who are not professional registered nurses but who are accountable to and work under the direct supervision of a professional registered nurse to implement specifically delegated patient care activities
- Evaluation of an individual state's/province's current nurse practice act to ensure that UAP job descriptions and delegated activities are consistent with established rules and regulations
- Written job descriptions that clearly delineate duties, responsibilities, qualifications, skills, and supervision of UAPS
- UAPs be readily identifiable by the patient as non-licensed
- Competence-based performance expectations and systems for ongoing performance appraisals

## AWHONN Clinical Position Statement: The Role of Unlicensed Assistive Personnel in the Nursing Care for Women and Newborns

- Orientation and training of UAPS, including didactic content, knowledge base evaluation, and clinical skills verification consistent with performance expectations and role responsibilities
- Clearly defined written parameters to ensure that all UAPs are supervised directly by and responsible to professional registered nurses; and
- Careful monitoring and evaluation of the impact of UAPs on adherence to care standards and patient outcomes (Adapted from American Association of Critical Care Nurses [AACNI], 1996)

Definitions:

Delegation

Transferring to a competent individual the authority to perform a selected nursing task in a selected situation. The professional registered nurse retains accountability for the delegation.

Accountability

Being responsible and answerable for actions and inactions of self or others in the context of delegation.

Supervision

The provision of guidance or direction, evaluation, and follow-up by the professional registered nurse for accomplishment of a nursing task delegated to UAPs.

(Adapted from the National Council of State Boards of Nursing, 1995)

In making the decision to delegate, the likely effects of the activity to be delegated should be assessed, using the following factors:

- potential for harm
- complexity of task
- problem solving and critical thinking required
- unpredictability of outcome
- level of care giver-patient interaction; and
- the practice setting (AACN, 1996)

Practice settings can include the inpatient setting, freestanding birthing center, surgery center, ambulatory care center, community health clinic, primary health care provider's office, and home care agency. The level of preparation, education, and competence of the person to whom the tasks are being delegated and how much supervision the professional registered nurse will be able to provide are important considerations. Some practice settings require much more autonomy on the part of the health care provider and allow less opportunity for supervision by the professional registered nurse than others. The knowledge base and clinical skills of the professional registered nurse provide the foundation for nursing assessments and diagnosis, critical thinking and decision making, outcome identification, planning, implementation, and evaluations that are requisite for high-quality outcomes for women and newborns. Distinguishing characteristics of the professional registered nurse are the type and amount of education, depth of knowledge, and critical thinking skills.

It is not appropriate to delegate nursing activities that comprise the core of the nursing process and require specialized knowledge, judgment, competence, and skill (ANA, 1994). These activities include, but are not limited to, performing initial patient assessments, making diagnoses, working with patients and families to identify outcomes and an appropriate plan of care, implementing the plan and evaluating the patient's progress or lack of progress toward achieving these goals. In addition, it is inappropriate to delegate any subsequent assessments or nursing interventions that require professional knowledge, judgment, and skill (ANA, 1994). Examples of nursing activities for women and newborns that should not be delegated are, but not limited to

- Telephone triage
- Initial assessment of women and newborns
- Application of fetal heart rate monitor
- Auscultation of fetal heart rate
- Initial and ongoing assessment of maternal-fetal status including auscultation and electronic fetal heart rate pattern interpretation
- Ongoing assessments of women receiving oxytocin infusion
- Ongoing assessments of pain management needs of women and newborns
- Ongoing assessments of women receiving regional analgesia/anesthesia
- Ongoing assessments of women who have complications of pregnancy
- Ongoing assessments of the progress of labor
- Management of the second stage of labor
- Circulation for vaginal or cesarean birth
- Initial assessment during the postpartum period after vaginal and cesarean birth
- Assessments required for discharge from postanesthesia care units
- Initial assessment of women and newborns during their post-surgical care
- Assigning APGAR scores

- Newborn identification
- Newborn assessments during the transition to extrauterine life
- Determining the plan of care based on nursing assessments
- Nursing interventions that require specialized knowledge, judgment, competence, and skill
- Discharge planning
- Patient teaching
- Parent teaching
- Evaluation of the outcome of nursing interventions.

When nursing activities or tasks are delegated to UAPs, professional registered nurses remain responsible and accountable for overall nursing care. Thus, patient assessment and diagnosis, outcome identification, care planning and implementation, and appropriately delegating tasks remain the responsibility of the professional registered nurse. The professional registered nurse is also accountable for ongoing supervision of UAPs and for evaluation of delegated activities, including patient outcomes. Some activities that are appropriate to delegate to UAPs include:

- Clerical duties
- Selected care tasks such as ambulation, feeding, mouth care and bathing
- Data gathering such as intake and output and vital signs

The responsibility for determining competence of UAPs who will perform delegated tasks and for evaluating each patient's clinical situation rests with the professional registered nurse. Delegated activities should be limited to clearly defined and thoroughly described repetitive tasks that do not require nursing judgments. Federal regulations, state nurse practice acts, board of nursing rules and regulations, and institutional guidelines must be followed any time nursing activities are delegated.

*Approved by the Executive Board, February 1997, September 2000.*

References
American Association of Critical Care Nurses. (1996, January/February). Clinical practice: Unlicensed assistive personnel. AACN News.

American Nurses Association. (1994). Registered professional nurses and unlicensed, assistive personnel. Washington, DC: Author.

National Council of State Boards of Nursing. (1995). Deleciation: Concepts and decision-making process. Chicago, IL: Author.

# Minimum RN Staffing in NICUs

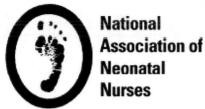

**National Association of Neonatal Nurses**

## NANN Position Statement #3009

### Introduction

External economic forces have led to disruptions in the classic regionalization plan for perinatal neonatal care. Intense competition for lucrative health care contracts has given hospitals a financial incentive to retain clients in their institutions or within their own systems, rather than transfer them to outside institutions (American Academy of Pediatrics, 1997). These economic pressures have prompted hospital administrators to redesign staffing patterns in an effort to cut operating costs.

The National Association of Neonatal Nurses (NANN) remains committed to promoting optimal, high-quality neonatal nursing care and advocating for newborns and their families. As part of this mission, the Association issues this position statement on absolute minimum professional nurse staffing in specialty care or subspecialty NICUs (Levels II, III, or variations of these levels). The delivery of safe and effective neonatal nursing care requires the assurance of a sufficient number of qualified registered nurses to attend to the emergent complex care needs of the patients.

Current nursing workloads in these critical care units are unprecedented as patient acuity, technology, and the scope of practice increases. Professional nursing resources must be sufficient to provide appropriate care based on the physiologic stability of individual patients to ensure delivery of a quality standard of nursing care-including parent education, bereavement care, and emergency response.

### Nurse Availability

In periods of increased census, more registered nurses are required. In periods of diminished census, these qualified registered nurses must remain immediately available to the neonatal specialty area. Additional nursing staff or on-call available staff resources must be appropriate to cover transport services;

outreach services; nursing resources shared or committed to other service areas, such as delivery room, admission, and observation areas, surgery, or radiology; and other nursing responsibilities specific to each unit.

During periods of decreased patient census or reduced patient acuity, an absolute minimum of two registered nurses are required to respond adequately to resuscitative emergencies; to assess emergent metabolic states such as hypoglycemia; and to manage cardiorespiratory emergencies such as mechanical ventilation or the decompression of a pneumothorax. Polin, Yoder, and Burg (1993) summarize the unique potential for sudden emergency intervention in the neonatal population, "No age group is more susceptible to asphyxia or is as frequently in need of resuscitation than the neonate".

Resuscitation occurrences are not confined to the delivery process. They can and do occur at any time during hospitalization. These events mandate the immediate availability of qualified personnel and equipment (Bloom & Cropley, 1998).

**Nurse-Patient Ratio**

During those periods when fewer than six intermediate patients or four intensive care neonatal patients are in the unit, it is NANN's position that at all times neonatal specialty care requires a minimum of two registered nurses with neonatal expertise and training.

This position statement supplements available staffing ratio recommendations such as those found in the American Academy of Pediatrics Guidelines for Perinatal Care (1997). These guidelines suggest a minimum staffing of one registered nurse for every two to three patients in intermediate care and one nurse for every one to two patients in intensive neonatal care. Administrative pressure may exist to reduce professional staff to one registered nurse or replace them with unlicensed personnel. NANN does not believe such staffing patterns provide for safe or adequate nursing care based on the needs of physiologically at risk or compromised neonatal patients. This position statement also supports the NANN Standards of Care for Neonatal Nursing Practice (NANN, 1998). NANN recognizes that minimum staffing ratios are sometimes set forth by the state. When there are state guidelines regarding staffing these must be followed.

## References

American Academy of Pediatrics. (1997). <u>Guidelines for perinatal care. 4th ed</u>. Elk Grove Village, IL: American Academy of Pediatrics and American College of Obstetricians and Gynecologists.

Bloom, R. S., & Cropley, C. (1998). American Academy of Pediatrics and American Heart Association. <u>Textbook of neonatal resuscitation</u>. Elk Grove Village, IL: American Academy of Pediatrics and American Heart Association.

National Association of Neonatal Nurses (NANN). (1998). <u>Standards of care for neonatal nursing practice</u>. Petaluma, CA: NANN.

Polin, R., Yoder, M., & Burg, F. (1993). <u>Workbook in practical neonatology. 2nd. Ed</u>. Philadelphia: Saunders.

---

*Approved, NANN Board of Directors, April 1999. Revised July, 2008.*

The National Association of Neonatal Nurses sets the standards for the neonatal nursing profession. Contact the association by phone at 800/451-3795, via e-mail at info@nann.org, and online at www.NANN.org.

# Bedside Registered Staff Nurse Shift Length, Fatigue, and Impact on Patient Safety

**NANN Position Statement #3044**

**NANN Board of Directors**
**August 28, 2008**

Nursing organizations across America have called upon nursing professionals to collectively establish safe-workplace strategies (Kenyon, Gluesing, White, Dunkel, & Burlingame, 2007). As the voice of neonatal nursing, the National Association of Neonatal Nurses (NANN) is issuing this position statement to enhance professional nursing practice and to encourage optimal care delivery to our tiny patients.

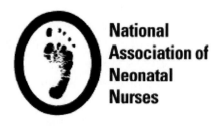

**National Association of Neonatal Nurses**

NANN Position Statement: Bedside Registered Staff Nurse Shift
Length, Fatigue, and Impact on Patient Safety

**Association Position**

The incidence and importance of fatigue are critical to every nurse's professional practice. NANN recommends education about fatigue be incorporated into nursing curriculum. NANN also recommends that all healthcare employers implement guidelines to minimize staff fatigue. Every RN should maintain awareness of his or her personal fatigue level because all RNs ultimately are responsible for their own practice.

**Background and Significance**

The effects of fatigue and sleep deprivation have been studied in a variety of nursing environments throughout the world. The ANA has established guidelines for nurses working in all areas of the nursing profession. The ANA position statement, "Assuring Patient Safety: The Employers' Role in Promoting Healthy Work Hours for Registered Nurses in All Roles and Settings," takes into account extensive research that links human fatigue with error for both nurses and nonnursing professionals such as truck drivers and airline pilots (ANA, 2006b). In addition, the ANA position statement details the responsibility of nurses to guard against working when fatigued.

In 2005, the Association of periOperative Registered Nurses (AORN) surveyed its members regarding on call hours and effects (Kenyon et al., 2007). Among respondents, 77% routinely took call, 68% said they had experienced sleep deprivation, 58% reported feeling unsafe while delivering patient care, and 13% reported making patient-care mistakes related to their fatigue (Kenyon et al.). Muecke (2005) published a study reviewing the impact of fatigue on nurses working in critical-care environments. Fatigue problems were categorized as a disturbance of circadian rhythm, physical and psychological issues, or disruption to family life. The study described sleep debt as a condition that occurs when a person experiences a decreased amount of sleep for multiple days.

The Minnesota Nurses Association (2007) found that nurses are 3 times more likely to make errors if they work shifts that are longer than 12 hours per day or 60 hours per week. In addition to being more prone to making medical errors, nurses who work longer shifts experience more neck, shoulder, and back injuries than nurses who work 8-hour shifts (Minnesota Nurses Association). The Arizona Nurses Association (2007) published research that indicates fatigue can cause physiological changes including impaired concentration, slowed reaction time, and reduced problem solving abilities.

Research on nursing fatigue clearly identifies the need to protect both nurses and patients from the effects of bedside nurses' fatigue and sleep deprivation. We concur with our colleagues who represent other nursing organizations and support the need for a healthcare culture that supports the prevention of fatigue and sleep deprivation for nurses, including those who, like our members, provide care for fragile patients in neonatal intensive care units.

## Recommendations

NANN recommends the following risk reduction strategies to decrease the fatigue and sleep deprivation nurses experience and to improve the safety of patients and nurses alike.

*For Employers and Nursing Managers/Directors:*
1. Promote a culture that recognizes nurse fatigue as an unacceptable risk (Kenyon et al., 2007).
2. Schedule sensibly. If an employee works both a day and night shift in the same week, it is recommended that he or she work the day shift first, followed by the night shift. After working a night shift, one day of rest is recommended before returning to the work environment (McGettrick & O'Neill, 2006).
3. Implement guidelines to limit the number of patient care hours a nurse can provide. Limitations for safe patient care include a maximum of 12 hours in a 24-hour period, and no more than 60 hours in a 7-day period (Institute of Medicine, 2004). In emergency situations, a staff nurse may be needed to work for a longer period of time, but this should be an exception due to unusual circumstances, such as severe weather.
4. Provide a sufficient number of off duty hours to allow an uninterrupted sleep cycle of at least 8 hours (Kenyon et al.).
5. Implement preplanned arrangements to relieve an RN if he or she is scheduled on-call for the next consecutive shift to allow time for a minimum of 8 hours of sleep. The number of on call shifts in a 7 day period should be incorporated into an RN's total scheduled hours (McGettrick & O'Neill, 2006).
6. Incorporate orientation to on-call as a part of new-hire orientation at all healthcare organizations (Kenyon et al.).
7. Consider permanent shift assignments; they may lessen fatigue effects (as opposed to rotating shifts; Muecke, 2005).

*For Bedside Registered Nurses:*
1. Nurses should uphold their ethical responsibility to arrive at work adequately rested and prepared to provide patient care.

2. Nurses need to consider that multiple workloads and work settings affect fatigue level (ANA, 2006a).
3. Bedside registered nurses should limit the number of hours they agree to work to a maximum of 12 hours in a 24 hour period (except in emergency situations), and to no more than 60 hours in a 7 day period (Kenyon et al.).

## Conclusions

The recommended strategies in this position statement should be considered in light of the specific circumstances of an individual institution. The resources available to an institution, the quality of those resources, and other factors will impact an institution's need and ability to adopt these recommendations.

## References

American Nurses Association. (2006a, December). *Assuring patient safety: Registered nurses' responsibility in all roles and settings to guard against working when fatigued.* Washington, DC: Author.

American Nurses Association. (2006b, December). *Assuring patient safety: The employers' role in promoting healthy nursing work hours for registered nurses in all roles and settings.* Washington, DC: Author.

Arizona Nurses Association. (2007). *Statement on nurse fatigue.* Tempe, AZ: Author.

Institute of Medicine. (2004). *Keeping patients safe: Transforming the work environment of nurses.* Washington, DC: National Academies Press.

Kenyon, T., Gluesing, R., White, K., Dunkel, W., & Burlingame, B. (2007). On call: Alert or unsafe? A report of the AORN On-Call Electronic Task Force. *AORN Journal*, 86(4), 630–639.

McGettrick, K., & O'Neill, M. (2006). Critical care nurses — Perceptions of 12-h shifts. *Nursing in Critical Care*, 11(4), 188–197.

Minnesota Nurses Association. (2007, January/February). #20 Nursing & fatigue. *Minnesota Nursing Accent*, 22–25.

Muecke, S. (2005). Effects of rotating night shifts: Literature review. *Journal of Advanced Nursing*, 50(4), 433–439.

## Bibliography

Blachowicz, E., & Letizia, M. (2006). The challenges of shift work. *MEDSURG Nursing*, 15(5), 274–280.

Dean, G., Scott, L., Rogers, A., Short, M., & Witt, C. (2006). Infants at risk: When nurse fatigue jeopardizes quality care. *Advances in Neonatal Care*, 6(3), 120–126.

Dewe, P. (1989). Stressor frequency, tension, tiredness and coping: Some measurement issues and a comparison among nursing groups. *Journal of Advanced Nursing*, 14, 308–320.

Emergency Nurses Association. (2003). *Emergency Nurses Association position statement: Staffing and productivity in the emergency care setting.* Des Plaines, IL: Author.

Halm, M., Peterson, M., Kendles, M., Sabo, J., Blalock, M., Braden, R., et al. (2005). Hospital nurse staffing and patient mortality, emotional exhaustion, and job dissatisfaction. *Clinical Nurse Specialist*, 19(5), 241–254.

Limiting the hours nurses should work. (2006, April–May). *Texas Nursing*, 6–7.

Nevada Nurses Association. (2007, May, June, and July). An overview of patient safety issues. *Nevada RNformation*, 4–6.

New York State Nurses Association. (2005). *Position statement on self care.* New York: Author.

Persson, M., & Martensson, J. (2006). Situations influencing habits in diet and exercise among nurses working night shift. *Journal of Nursing Management*, 14(5), 414–423.

Richardson, A., Turnock, C., Harris, L., Finley, A., & Carson, S. (2007). A study examining the impact of 12-hour shifts on a critical care staff. *Journal of Nursing Management*, 15(8), 838–846.

Rogers, A. (2004). The working hours of hospital staff nurses and patient safety. *Health Affairs*, 23(4), 202–212.

Sabo, B. (2006). Compassion fatigue and nursing work: Can we accurately capture the consequences of caring work? *International Journal of Nursing Practice*, 12, 136–142.

Seki, Y., & Yamazaki, Y. (2006). Effects of working conditions on intravenous medication errors in a Japanese hospital. *Journal of Nursing Management*, 14(2), 128–139.

Thomas, M. (2005). Study examines working hours and feelings of fatigue by reported nurses. *Texas Board of Nursing Bulletin*, 36(4), 2–3.

Winwood, P., & Lushington, K. (2006). Disentangling the effects of psychological and physical work demands on sleep, recovery and maladaptive chronic stress outcomes within a large sample of Australian nurses. *Journal of Advanced Nursing*, 56(6), 679–689.

Winwood, P., Winefield, A., & Lushington, K. (2006). Work-related fatigue and recovery: The contribution of age, domestic responsibilities and shiftwork. *Journal of Advanced Nursing*, 56(4), 438–449.

Wisconsin Nursing Coalition, & Wisconsin Nurses Association. (2007, July). Nurse fatigue and patient safety research and recommendations.

NANN Position Statement: Bedside Registered Staff Nurse Shift
Length, Fatigue, and Impact on Patient Safety

*Stat Bulletin*, 3–4.

---

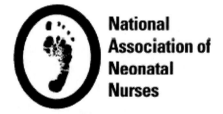

**National
Association of
Neonatal
Nurses**

# Glossary of Legal Terms

**Affidavit**      A written statement made or taken under oath before an officer of the court or a notary public or other authorized to act.

**Allegation**      In pleading, an assertion of fact.

**Arbitration**      The conducting of a trial in front of one or more arbitrators (usually malpractice attorneys or retired judges) who act in place of the judge and jury, and decide the case.

**Attest**      To affirm as true.

**Defendant**      The person against whom the suit is brought.

**Deposition**      A method of pretrial discovery that consists of a statement of a witness under oath taken in question and answer form as it would in court, with opportunity given to the adversary to be present and to cross-examine the witness.

**Discovery**      Modern pretrial procedure by which one party gains vital information concerning the case held by the adverse party, including depositions and interrogatories.

**Evidence**      All means by which any alleged matter of fact is established or disproved.

**Expert Witness**      One who possesses special knowledge, skills, and experience in a specific area and whose testimony as to his or her opinion is admissible as evidence.

**Immunity**      Protection from being sued.

**Interrogatories**      A method of pretrial discovery in which written questions are proposed by one party and served on the adversary party; written replies must be made under oath. Interrogatories can only be served to the parties named in the action.

**Liability**      An obligation one has incurred or might incur through any act or failure to act, responsibility for conduct falling below a certain standard, which is the cause of the plaintiff's injury.

**Malpractice**      Professional misconduct, improper discharge of professional duties, or a failure to meet the standard of care by a professional that results in harm to another.

**Negligence**      Failure to act as an ordinary prudent person; conduct contrary to that of a reasonable person under specific circumstances.

**Plaintiff**      The person who brings a civil suit seeking damages or legal relief.

| | |
|---|---|
| **Standard of Care** | The conduct that a prudent nurse with similar education, training, and experience would undertake in similar circumstances; the standard to which the defendant's conduct is compared to ascertain negligence. |
| **Statute of Limitations** | A legal limit on the time one has to file a suit in civil matters, usually measured from the time the wrong was or should have been discovered. |
| **Subpoena** | A court order compelling the appearance of a witness at a judicial proceeding. |

Reference: Rostant, D. & Cady, R. (1999). <u>Liability issues in perinatal nursing</u>. Lippincott: Philadelphia.